S0-AQJ-500

Clinical Judgment in Community Health Nursing

Clinical Judgment in Community Health Nursing

A Workbook for Group and Self-Paced Learning

Michele A. Hadeka, R.N., M.S.
Associate Professor, Community Health Nursing
School of Nursing
The University of Vermont

Little, Brown and Company
Boston   Toronto

Library of Congress Cataloging-in-Publication Data

Hadeka, Michele A.
  Clinical judgment in community health nursing.

  Includes index.
  1. Community health nursing—Problems, exercises, etc.
2. Community health nursing—Programmed instruction.
I. Title. [DNLM: 1. Community Health Nursing—programmed
instruction. WY 18 H128c]
RT98.H33   1986   610.73'43   86–2865
ISBN 0–316–33713–7

Copyright © 1987 by Michele A. Hadeka

All rights reserved. No part of this book may be reproduced in any form
or by any electronic or mechanical means including information stor-
age and retrieval systems without permission in writing from the publisher except by a reviewer who may quote brief passages in a review.

Library of Congress Catalog Card No. 86–2865

ISBN 0-316-33713-7

9 8 7 6 5 4 3 2 1

MV

Published simultaneously in Canada
by Little, Brown and Company (Canada) Limited
Printed in the United States of America

Credits

pp. 55–58, 67–69. From M. A. Hadeka and J. Sutherland, "Community Assessment" (unpublished paper, 1977). Used by permission of the authors.

pp. 61–62. Reprinted with permission of the present publisher, Jones and Bart-
lett Publishers, Inc., from S. E. Archer and R. P. Fleshman, *Community Health
Nursing*, 2d ed., Wadsworth Health Sciences, © 1979, p. 230, and *Community
Health Nursing*, 3d ed., Wadsworth Health Sciences, © 1985, pp. 100, 102, 104.

pp. 127, 220–221. From S. L. Shamansky and C. L. Clausen, "Levels of Prevention: Examination of the Concept." Copyright © 1980, American Journal of
Nursing Company. Excerpted with permission from *Nursing Outlook*, Febru-
ary 1980, Vol. 28, No. 2, pp. 104–108.

pp. 147–148. From I. M. Rosenstock, "Historical Origins of the Health Belief
Model," in M. H. Becker, ed., *The Health Belief Model and Personal Health Behavior* (Thorofare, NJ: Slack, 1974), pp. 1–8. Reprinted by permission.

pp. 152–153. From J. Berkenfield and J. Schwartz, "Nutrition intervention in the
community—the 'WIC' program," *The New England Journal of Medicine*
302(10):579–581, 1980. Reprinted by permission.

To Peter Salzberg, my husband, friend, and mentor, who has encouraged my creativity and challenged me to take risks.

To Faith Emerson and Mary Julia Cronin, my respected colleagues, who supported me in this endeavor from its inception.

To Adolph and Eileen Hadeka, my parents, with love.

INTRODUCTION
What This Workbook Is About

Dear Students and Community Health Nurses:

Clinical Judgment in Community Health Nursing: A Workbook for Group and Self-Paced Learning is a workbook written for you. My purpose is to help you apply the nursing process when problem solving and also to apply your basic nursing knowledge in a variety of community health settings.

In my experience at the University of Vermont I have seen students, and at times staff nurses, become frustrated deciding how to handle a situation on a home visit or in a school health room when the clinical instructor or another nurse was not at hand. Yet, when reviewing the situation later with the instructor or a supervisor, the student or staff nurse has been able to solve the problem by applying the nursing process, dissecting the situation, and solving one aspect of it at a time.

I have also seen students and staff nurses become frustrated as they find how the concept of community applies to their roles in working with individual clients and families in community agencies. Community health nursing does entail more than focusing on the individual and family—it requires that we focus on the health and welfare of the larger community by working with communities as well as groups and aggregates. In the clinical setting, students and staff generally do not see the nursing role with this broader community focus because it occurs primarily at supervisory and administrative levels.

To assist students and staff with these frustrations I have developed this workbook of clinical situations to involve you in solving problems with individual clients and families similar to difficulties you may encounter in any clinical area. I have also included situations focused on the aggregate and community similar to those you may encounter as a staff nurse working in a community agency.

The workbook is composed of fifteen situations, each originating in one of four community health nursing settings: Home Health Agency/VNA, School Health, Maternal-Child Health, and Occupational Health. Nine of the situations are designed for you to complete by yourself, and six are to be completed by you in group discussion with other nursing students and a community health clinical instructor, in an in-service session for staff and supervisors, or in a combination of these. In each of the four sections, the first situations are relatively uncomplicated; subsequent situations are increasingly complex.

As you are completing the situations, you may ask at times, "Could this really happen?" Rest assured that it has. The situations I have written are all based upon real individuals, families, and communities, some with minor alterations. Names and other identifying characteristics have been changed.

When completing the self-paced situations:

1. Read the information.
2. Write your answer.
3. Proceed to the appropriate page to compare your answers.
4. Proceed to the next step.

When completing the group discussion situations:

1. Read the information.
2. Write your answer.
3. Participate in group discussion—it's fun!
4. Record and analyze new information the clinical instructor gives you.
5. Write your answer.
6. Participate in group discussion.

I strongly encourage you to use the work space provided to *write your own answers* in all the situations in order to learn from them. You need to make a decision, a commitment: Write what you think and support your thoughts with a rationale. When you don't write your answers, several thoughts may be going through your mind and you may remain uncommitted to any one of them. You then read the suggested answer or hear the group discussion and say to yourself, "That's just what I was thinking!" If in fact you had written an answer, it might have been quite different.

When completing the self-paced situations, avoid jumping immediately to the answers; this shortcut defeats the purpose of the exercise and leaves you with an inaccurate representation of how you would have managed the situation.

On occasion you will find that no one answer is right. In most clinical situations there may be more than one way to solve a problem. Often two nurses will agree on what the results of a situation should or could be, but the same two may disagree on how to proceed to achieve the desired results. At times, your answers may be somewhat different from those suggested. That's okay *if* you can support your answer with a solid rationale based upon nursing theory and the basic sciences.

If you find that your answers consistently differ greatly from those suggested, take time to work with your community health instructor or your nursing supervisor and find out why.

Nursing students at the University of Vermont have enjoyed doing these situations. I have been impressed by their interest and the quality of their answers. I hope you too will find the situations interesting and challenging. My fervent hope is that you will learn not only about the gaps in your knowledge but also about the strengths. Good luck!

Sincerely,

Michele A. Hadeka

Michele A. Hadeka, R.N., M.S.
Associate Professor, Community Health Nursing
School of Nursing
The University of Vermont
Burlington, Vermont

Acknowledgments

There are many community health nurses, colleagues, students, clients, family members, and friends who have made this book possible. I thank each and every one of them for their interest, enthusiasm, and support.

I would like to thank all those who reviewed the manuscript: Fran Whited, Texas Woman's University; Linda Lee Daniel, University of Michigan; Joan Baldwin, Idaho State University; Barbara Spradley, University of Minnesota; and Joan Mulligan, University of Wisconsin, Madison.

A special thank-you goes to the women who have played major roles in the production of this book: my typist, Barbara La-Duke; my editor, Ann West; and Barbara Breese at Little, Brown and Company.

CONTENTS

Clinical Judgment in Community Health Nursing

Notice

The indications and dosages of all drugs in this book have been recommended in the medical literature and conform to the practices of the general medical community. The medications described do not necessarily have specific approval by the Food and Drug Administration for use in the diseases and dosages for which they are recommended. The package insert for each drug should be consulted for use and dosage as approved by the FDA. Because standards for usage change, it is advisable to keep abreast of revised recommendations, particularly those concerning new drugs.

PART I

Home Health Agency/VNA

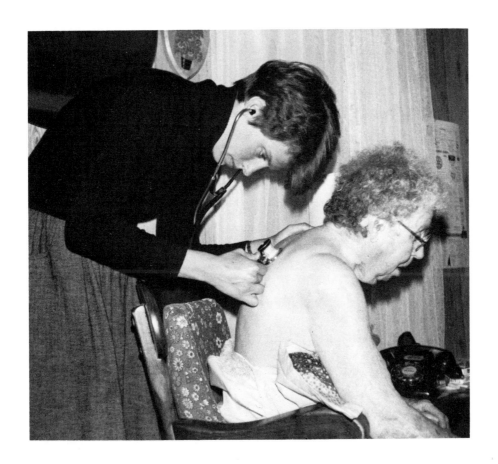

⋙⋙⋘ SITUATION 1 ⋙⋙⋘
The Home Visit:
Application of Principles
⋙⋙ (Group Discussion) ⋙⋙

Introduction to all sections: It is Wednesday morning. Upon your arrival at the home health agency, you find a new referral on your desk from a local physician. You are being asked to make a home visit to evaluate Mrs. Wright, a 78-year-old woman who arrived five days ago from a distant state with her 75-year-old husband to stay indefinitely at her granddaughter's home. The referral states that the couple's arrival was unexpected and that the granddaughter is apprehensive about caring for them. (A niece who had been overseeing their care, finances, etc., is now acutely ill and can no longer handle this responsibility.)

Mrs. Wright has a history of degenerative joint disease in her right hip and has been unable to ambulate for three years. She is confined to bed. Mrs. Wright has no other known medical problems.

SECTION 1.1

In order to make an effective therapeutic home visit to this family you need to have a clear understanding of what a therapeutic home visit entails.

In the work space provided:

    a. Write a definition for a therapeutic home visit.
    b. Based upon your definition, what level of prevention would you anticipate practicing—primary, secondary, or tertiary?

Student Work Space _____

3

SECTION 1.2

When you arrive at the granddaughter's home to evaluate Mrs. Wright, the granddaughter greets you at the front door. She tells you that her *grandfather,* Mr. Wright, has not had a bowel movement since he arrived at her home. He was seen by her family physician yesterday. The physician ordered two disposable enemas and told the granddaughter you would give them when you came to see Mrs. Wright. The granddaughter hands you the disposable enemas.

In the work space provided, answer the following:

Should you provide direct care for *Mr. Wright?* If no, why? If yes, why? How?

Student Work Space

SECTION 1.3

After being introduced to Mrs. Wright, you spend the next 1½ hours gathering a nursing history and doing a comprehensive physical assessment on Mrs. Wright. In brief, your assessment reveals the following:

Her skin color is pale; lips are pale, conjunctiva are pink. She is alert and oriented to person, place, and time. Her B/P is 110/80, pulse 82 and regular, respirations 22 and even. Her lungs are clear. Her peripheral circulation is good, i.e., radial, pedal, and popliteal pulses are present, all extremities are warm to the touch, and there is no evidence of edema. She says she takes no prescribed medications or over-the-counter drugs.

Mrs. Wright moves well in bed with minimal assistance. She can transfer on and off a bedpan easily. She has good use of her arms with full range of motion. She can sit up in bed if propped with pillows.

Mrs. Wright has limited range of motion in both legs, i.e., she can raise each leg only to a 15° angle, but she can bend both knees easily. Both feet are plantar-flexed; minimal ankle movement is possible. The granddaughter says Mrs. Wright was evaluated for a hip replacement at a large medical center last year but was advised against surgery because of the extent of the hip degeneration and her age.

Based upon your assessment of Mrs. Wright:

    a. What would be your overall goal for her?

    b. Would other agency services be appropriate for her?
       If no, stop here.
       If yes, identify the services you think would be appropriate and provide a brief description of what each service could offer Mrs. Wright.

Student Work Space

SECTION 1.4

In your discussion with Mrs. Wright she tells you that ever since she has been confined to bed her husband has assisted her with her personal care. Now that they have moved into the granddaughter's home, there seems to be some uncertainty about who should be responsible for Mrs. Wright's care. Mr. Wright wants to maintain his role, but the granddaughter feels it is now her role.

In the work space provided:

    a. Identify who you think should be responsible for Mrs. Wright's personal care. State your rationale.
    b. State how you would present your recommendation regarding Mrs. Wright's care to the couple/family.

Student Work Space

SECTION 1.5

As your visit concludes, you feel good about the plan you have developed with the couple and the granddaughter.

Before leaving, you take the granddaughter aside to ask about the impact of this unexpected visit (with all of its responsibilities) on her and her family. The granddaughter tells you that she doesn't want to upset her grandparents, but she is having serious marital problems and, until their arrival, was planning to leave her husband.

In the work space provided, answer the following:

    a. Will this information affect your plans? If no, why? If yes, how?
    b. Is involvement in the granddaughter's problems part of your role? If no, why? If yes, how?

Student Work Space

Suggested Reading

Hadeka, M. (1983). Why don't nurses use contracts? *Vermont Registered Nurse*, January 1983, 11–15.

Humphrey, P., Hewitt, D. W., & Craven, R. F. (1983). Adaptation through the life cycle. In W. J. Phipps, B. C. Long, & N. F. Woods (Eds.). *Medical-surgical nursing.* (2d ed.) St. Louis: Mosby (pp. 202–246).

Keeling, B. L. (1978). Making the most of the first home visit. *Nursing '78* 8(24): 24–25.

Lockhart, C. A. (1979). Family-focused community health nursing services in the home. In S. E. Archer & R. P. Fleshman (Eds.). *Community health nursing.* (2d ed.) Belmont, CA: Wadsworth (pp. 152–175).

Malasanos, L., Barkauskas, V., Moss, M., & Stoltenberg-Allen, K. (1981). *Health assessment.* St. Louis: Mosby.

Mitchell, P. H. (1983). Adaptation, stress and coping. In W. J. Phipps, B. C. Long, & N. F. Woods (Eds.). *Medical-surgical nursing.* (2d ed.) St. Louis: Mosby (pp. 161–169).

Price, J. L., & Braden, C. (1978). The reality in home visits. *American Journal of Nursing* 78: 1536–1538.

Shamansky, S. L., & Clausen, C. L. (1980). Levels of prevention: Examination of the concept. *Nursing Outlook* 28(2): 104–108.

Spradley, B. W. (1985). *Community health nursing: Concepts and practice.* (2d ed.) Boston: Little, Brown.

Wiles, E. (1984). Home health care nursing. In M. Stanhope & J. Lancaster (Eds.). *Community health nursing.* St. Louis: Mosby (pp. 780–801).

SITUATION 2
Who Is Right, Anyway?
(Self-Paced)

SECTION 2.1

It is a Wednesday in mid-July. Many of the staff members in the home health agency are taking summer vacations. Joyce, your good friend and the staff nurse with whom you share an office, will be going on vacation next week. You have agreed to cover some clients in her caseload while she is away. Joyce has given you a verbal summary on each client. You have reviewed their records and believe you have a good understanding of how each client is progressing.

There is one elderly woman, Mrs. Thomas, who has an ulcer on her right ankle which is healing poorly. She has daily dressing changes. Joyce asks you to make a joint visit with her today so that she can demonstrate the dressing protocol. She thinks this is a good approach because Mrs. Thomas adapts poorly to change, and a joint visit may reduce her concerns.

Figure 1 is Joyce's sketch of the appearance, location, and measurements of the ulcer. Including such a sketch in a patient's record is an excellent technique that enables comparison by other nurses caring for the client.

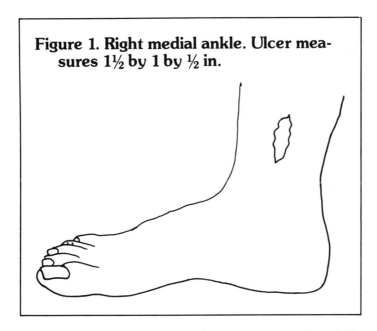

Figure 1. Right medial ankle. Ulcer measures 1½ by 1 by ½ in.

During the visit, Joyce demonstrates her dressing protocol as follows:

1. She asks Mrs. Thomas to lie down on her bed and elevate her legs; she places a protective padding on the bed under Mrs. Thomas's leg.
2. She loosens the tape which is securing all four sides of the dressing.
3. She picks up the foul-smelling dressing and discards it in the waste-paper basket near the bed. You now have a clear view of the ankle ulcer; it is approximately 1½ by 1 by ½ in. It has a foul odor.

4. Joyce then opens a package of sterile 4-by-4-in. gauze sponges; she takes them into the adjoining bathroom and moistens them with tap water.
5. She returns to the bedside and scrubs the open wound with a moist 4 by 4 to loosen a small amount of eschar present.
6. She discards the 4 by 4 in the wastepaper basket near the bed.
7. She opens two packages of 4 by 4 gauze sponges, places them over the ulcer, and tapes all four sides of the dressing.

In the work space provided:

a. State whether or not you agree with Joyce's dressing protocol.
b. State rationale supporting your opinion.

If your opinion differs from Joyce's:

c. Is there additional equipment you would like? If so, what?
d. Briefly outline your protocol.

Student Work Space

Turn to the following pages to compare your answers.
a. agree/disagree with protocol – p. 12
b. rationale – p. 13
c. additional equipment – p. 14
d. your protocol – p. 15

SECTION 2.2

As you return to the office with Joyce, she asks you if you are comfortable with Mrs. Thomas's dressing protocol.

In the work space provided:

a. What do you tell her?
b. If you disagree with the protocol, how do you present your opinion without offending her?
c. How do you think this problem can be resolved?

Student Work Space

Turn to the following pages to compare your answers.
a. what you tell her – p. 16
b. your opinion – p. 17
c. resolving the problem – p. 17

SECTION 2.3

As a student nurse in community health confronted with a situation in which you disagree with a staff nurse, how would you approach the problem?

In the work space provided:

a. State your opinion.
b. Support your opinion with rationale.

Student Work Space

Turn to the following pages to compare your answers.
a. your opinion – p. 18
b. rationale – p. 18

SECTION 2.4 _____

OR

As a staff nurse in community health, how would you respond to a student who tells you your technique is faulty?

In the work space provided:

a. State how you think you would respond.

Student Work Space_____

Turn to the following page to compare your answer.
a. your response – p. 19

ANSWERS TO SECTION 2.1 _____

a. Agree/disagree with Joyce's protocol

b. Rationale supporting opinion

If you agree with Joyce's protocol, perhaps rereading the protocol would be wise. When rereading the protocol, look for breaks in aseptic technique.

If you agree that Joyce is correct in not approaching this dressing change as a "sterile" procedure, you may be basing your rationale on the concept of medical asepsis or "clean" technique. However, does the concept of medical asepsis or "clean" technique apply here? Review these definitions:

Surgical Asepsis (Sterile Technique) (Murray & Valentine, 1981, p. 144). This term is used when dealing with an area that may or may not be sterile. The goal is to avoid introducing any new organisms to the area. Therefore, the measures involved in sterile technique are those that will protect the area from anything in the environment that is not sterile. This technique is used whenever the first line of defense has been broken, as from a wound, surgical incision, or needle prick or when entering any usually sterile cavity in the body such as the urinary bladder.

Medical Asepsis (Clean Technique) (Murray & Valentine, 1981, p. 144). When working with an area of the body that is usually not sterile or with an intact line of defense, sterile technique is not necessary, and measures involved in medical asepsis are used. Clean technique would be used in the mouth or to put a tube from the nose to the stomach; to give an enema; or to apply a hot pack to a swollen area.

As you read the definitions, it becomes clear that medical asepsis is not appropriate in this situation and that surgical asepsis is.

Ideally, the outcome you would like for Mrs. Thomas is to have her leg ulcer heal. What are the chances of its healing without using sterile technique?

If you disagree with Joyce's protocol, congratulations! In reviewing her technique, violations of sterile technique can be identified in almost every step.

For example	*Rationale*
1. Joyce does not wash her hands at any time during the dressing change.	1. Whether a procedure is "sterile" or "clean," hand washing is essential. The skin harbors many microorganisms which the individual may be resistant to, but if resistance is altered, the microorganisms may become pathogens (Leslie & Pakatar, 1980). Mrs. Thomas has an open wound (a portal of entry); microorganisms introduced into her wound through direct or indirect contact could easily become pathogens. All wounds are at risk for infection (Leslie & Pakatar, 1980). People become immune to their own "normal" microorganisms, i.e., organisms with which they have frequent contact and have developed a defense against. They may not be immune to those introduced by others (Murray & Valentine, 1981).
2. Joyce does not use gloves during the dressing change.	2. Clean gloves protect the nurse from the environment and should be used in removing the soiled dressing. Sterile gloves are used to decrease the transfer of microorganisms from the environment to the wound; sterile gloves should be used when cleansing the wound and applying a new dressing (Leslie & Pakatar, 1980).
3. Joyce moves around the wound several times and does not organize herself or her equipment.	3. Additional movement around the open wound increases the chances that microorganisms will be transferred through direct or indirect contact.
4. Joyce handles the soiled dressing and disposes of the dressing improperly.	4. Microorganisms are transferred through moist or wet surfaces in a capillary action (Murray & Valentine, 1981), e.g., through the dressing to the nurse's hands. Throwing soiled dressings in an open wastebasket is conducive to spread of the microorganisms by insects, pets, or contact with the individual emptying the basket. The dressings and 4 by 4's used for cleansing the wound should be placed in a paper bag that can be

closed, or they should be wrapped in a newspaper, placed in a waterproof container such as a plastic bag, and sealed or burned.

5. Joyce cleanses the wound with a 4 by 4 and tap water held in her hand.

5. The same principles of microorganism transfer discussed above under hand washing apply here. In addition, the solution used, i.e., tap water, is not sterile. Sterilization renders objects and areas free from all microorganisms (Feeley, Shine, & Sloboda, 1980).

6. Joyce uses contaminated equipment.

6. The principles of microorganism transfer also apply here, as Joyce touches all equipment without hand washing, e.g., handling a sterile dressing. In addition, she does not prepare her equipment through sterilization, e.g., basin, forceps, water. Sterilization renders objects and areas free from all microorganisms (Feeley et al., 1980).

7. Joyce uses adhesive tape on a precarious site.

7. The skin surrounding the wound is susceptible to breakdown as a result of peripheral vascular disease. If skin breakdown occurs, another portal of entry has been established.

Aspects of the procedure that Joyce does correctly	*Rationale*
1. Joyce has the client lie down.	1. Facilitates circulation and the dressing change.
2. Joyce places a protective padding between the client's leg and bed.	2. Protects the client's bed.

c. **Equipment needed**

*1 large pan (stainless steel or aluminum) for sterilizing basin and forceps
1 small basin (stainless steel or aluminum)
1 forceps
1 pair clean gloves

1 pair sterile gloves
3 packages sterile 4 by 4's
1 roll Kerlix or Kling
1 roll adhesive tape
1 plastic or paper bag or newspaper
water

*Some individuals may choose to use only one pan instead of two.

Note: The basin, forceps, and water can be sterilized by the nurse on arriving at the client's home or by the client before the nurse arrives. Boiling time should be at least *10 minutes* and timed from when the water begins to boil (Leslie & Pakatar, 1980). The forceps/hemostat should be placed in the basin for sterilizing to facilitate easy transfer of the sterile equipment to the bedside.

Please Note: The following protocol is *suggested.* If your protocol varies but adheres to the principles of aseptic technique, good for you!

d. Suggested protocol for dressing change

Protocol	*Rationale*
1. Position Mrs. Thomas lying down.	1. Facilitates circulation, dressing change.
2. Wash hands; use running water, emulsifying agent, and friction. Dry hands thoroughly.	2. Hand washing decreases transfer of microorganisms (Leslie & Pakatar, 1980).
3. Place dry equipment, i.e., gloves, 4 by 4's, etc., within easy reach.	3. Organization will decrease the need to move around the open wound.
4. Transport freshly sterilized equipment and place within easy reach. (To transport the equipment without contaminating it, pour the excess water from the large sterilizing pan. Allow the pan and its contents to cool. Reach into the pan and remove the smaller pan, *touching only the outside* of the pan. The forceps should be inside; pour off all but about 100 cc of excess water without dislodging the forceps.)	4. Sterilization renders areas and objects free of microorganisms (Feeley et al., 1980). Microorganisms are transferred by direct/indirect contact (Murray & Valentine, 1981). Touching only the outside of the basin avoids direct contact with the inside and its contents.
5. Gently remove tape from sides of dressing.	5. The use of tape should be questioned because poor peripheral circulation is already a problem, as evidenced by the ulcer. Repeated application of tape can cause further breakdown.
6. Put on clean gloves.	6. Microorganisms are transferred through moist or wet surfaces in a capillary action (Murray & Valentine, 1981); the gloves act as a barrier between the dressing and the nurse.
7. Remove old dressing; dispose of soiled dressing and gloves in paper/plastic bag/newspaper.	7. Microorganisms are transferred by direct/indirect contact (Murray & Valentine, 1981).
8. Open 3 packages of 4 by 4's, leaving 2 packages on their wrappers. Drop the third into the sterile water in the sterile basin.	8. Two packages are open and will be easily accessible once sterile gloves are put on. The third package of 4 by 4's will be ready for cleansing the wound.
9. Put on sterile gloves.	9. Gloves act as a barrier be-

10. Reach into the sterile basin and pick up the forceps. Use the forceps to pick up the moistened 4 by 4's and . . .
11. Cleanse the wound gently.

12. Dispose of the moistened 4 by 4 in the bag or newspaper.

13. Let wound air dry.

14. With gloved hand pick up dry, sterile 4 by 4's and cover the wound.
15. Hold dressing in place and wrap (ankle to foot) dressing with Kling or Kerlix. Place tape on end of Kerlix to hold in place.
16. Cleanse basin and forceps thoroughly with water, emulsifying agent, and friction.
17. Remove gloves and dispose of in plastic bag.

18. Rewash your own hands.

tween sterile field and nurse (Leslie & Pakatar, 1980).
10. Gloves act as a barrier between sterile field and nurse (Leslie & Pakatar, 1980).

11. Removes debris and stimulates circulation to the area.
12. Microorganisms are transferred through a capillary action (Murray & Valentine, 1981).
13. Microorganisms prefer warm, moist areas for growth.
14. Sterile glove acts as a barrier between sterile 4 by 4's and the nurse's hand.
15. Securing the dressing in place with Kerlix/Kling decreases the chance of damaging skin integrity.

16. Microorganisms are transferred by direct/indirect contact (Murray & Valentine, 1981).
17. Microorganisms are transferred by direct/indirect contact (Murray & Valentine, 1981).
18. Microorganisms are transferred by direct/indirect contact (Murray & Valentine, 1981).

ANSWERS TO SECTION 2.2

a. What do you tell Joyce?

In a situation like this one, where you know that another nurse's technique is faulty and where you will be assuming responsibility for the client's care, as an accountable professional you have to speak up. (Even if you were not assuming responsibility for the client's care, you still should discuss Joyce's technique with her.) You have identified basic principles which have been violated, and they need to be acknowledged. It is possible that the breaks in technique have delayed wound healing.

If in this situation Joyce had not asked for your critique, you would still need to volunteer it. The violation of principles must be acknowledged.

However, *how* you approach Joyce will determine whether her response will be positive or negative.

b. How do you present your opinion without offending Joyce?

Presenting your opinion to Joyce is obviously difficult. As her friend and colleague you are naturally concerned about hurting her feelings. In this situation, it is important to understand the difference between assertive behavior and aggressive behavior. Assertive nurses can address difficult situations, communicating their feelings effectively without humiliating or hurting the other individual. Assertive nurses are goal and action oriented but do not pursue goals at the expense of others. They express their feelings in an honest and genuine fashion with no intention of hurting the other person (Baer, 1976; Pointer & Lancaster, 1984).

An assertive technique that would be useful in this situation with Joyce is the use of "I" statements. For example:

> "I feel uncomfortable . . ."
> "I feel uneasy . . ."
> "I am concerned about . . ."

Let her know what you are uncomfortable, uneasy, and/or concerned about. The basis of the "I" statement is that the individual receiving the message (Joyce) is approached in a nonaccusatory fashion and the individual speaking is assuming responsibility for what is being said. "I" statements are not easy; they require some forethought (Baer, 1976; Pointer & Lancaster, 1984).

As individuals we are much more familiar with "You" statements such as:

> "You're doing it all wrong . . ."
> "Don't you realize what you're doing . . ."
> "Your technique needs improvement . . ."

Unfortunately, these statements are accusatory in nature and tend to make the individual receiving the message feel angry, hurt, or defensive. "You" statements tend to be aggressive. Aggressive nurses achieve their own goals at any cost, often at the expense of others (Baer, 1976; Pointer & Lancaster, 1984).

Take time to listen to how others approach you and how you approach others. Are there lots of "You" statements? Are there many "I" statements?

c. How do you think this problem can be resolved?

If you approach the problem as one that you and Joyce can work out together, she is more likely to listen to what you have to say. You can:

1. Explain your concern(s) using "I" statements.
2. Ask her to tell you how she arrived at her protocol. As she reviews the steps, you will have an opportunity to point out specific procedures that seem to you to violate the principles of aseptic technique. For example, you might say, "But tap water isn't sterile. Aren't we running the risk that microorganisms will be transferred to the wound?"
3. Give her time to respond to your concerns.

There are several options if she's willing to learn. Remember to apply the principles of teaching and learning as described on pages 133–136.

1. Practice/demonstrate with her before a revisit.
2. Revisit with her and show her and the client your protocol. Have Joyce explain the change in protocol to the client.

3. Revisit with her and let her walk through your protocol. Have Joyce explain the change in protocol to the client.
4. Help her to problem-solve the dressing change, once she understands the principles of microorganism transfer.

Of the above options, helping Joyce to problem-solve is an excellent choice. In the process of problem solving, you (Wykle, 1983):

1. Remain open, sensitive to her needs, and nonjudgmental regarding her questions.
2. Help her identify specifically what the problem is, i.e., failure to observe the principles of aseptic technique, not wanting to take time to do the dressing correctly, etc. Discuss with her what to say to Mrs. Thomas about the change in procedure. This should be dealt with whether Mrs. Thomas asks or not. For example, "Joyce and I have discussed your ulcer care and have arrived at some techniques we think will help it to heal."
3. Review with her the principles of microorganism transfer.
4. Give her time to question, explore, think.
5. Help her identify consequences of her technique.
6. Help her identify alternatives to her present technique which will not violate principles of aseptic technique.
7. Provide her with positive reinforcement as she proceeds with problem solving.

If Joyce is not willing to learn:

1. Establish your own protocol with the client, explaining to the client that you have discussed her ulcer care with Joyce and will be changing the routine and using some techniques you think will help. Involve the client in the process, enlisting her help in preparing the sterile basin and forceps/hemostat.
2. Encourage Joyce to seek consultation from the nursing supervisor through an informal conference. Let her know you are willing to participate.
3. If Joyce chooses not to seek consultation from the supervisor, it is your responsibility to discuss the situation with the supervisor. Tell Joyce what you are going to do, and explain your rationale, i.e., professional responsibility to protect the patient.

ANSWERS TO SECTION 2.3

a. As a student nurse in community health confronted with a situation in which you disagree with a staff nurse, how would you approach the problem?

b. Rationale

All too often student nurses are placed in situations with staff nurses similar to this. Student nurses generally respond in one of two ways:

1. They compromise their values and follow the staff nurse's example because they "do not want to offend" the staff nurse (nonassertive behavior).

2. They argue with and alienate the staff nurse (aggressive behavior).

As a general rule, the above approaches will produce the same results each time. As a student nurse you do have a right to your opinion, and you have the responsibility to support your opinion with solid, well-thought-through rationale.

The *key*, again, is *how* you approach the staff nurse. The discussion of assertive behavior on page 17 with Joyce applies here as well. Using "I" statements as suggested is again an excellent way to let the staff nurse know what you are feeling about the situation.

Students who have taken the time to think about using assertive techniques such as "I" statements with staff nurses (and others) have been pleasantly surprised with the results.

If the staff nurse does not respond positively, i.e., is unwilling to discuss your concerns or unwilling to learn, you need to seek guidance from your clinical instructor. Your clinical instructor may help you identify ways to approach the staff nurse or may take an active role and hold an informal discussion with you and the staff nurse.

ANSWERS TO SECTION 2.4

a. State how you think you would respond.

The staff nurse's response to a criticism/critique by a student can be either positive or negative.

A negative response, i.e., angry or defensive, may result in further negative communication with the student. Such a response can leave both the staff nurse and the student feeling uncomfortable about the interaction and may leave the situation unresolved.

A positive response, i.e., nondefensive, open, willing to discuss the situation, is likely to result in positive interaction between the staff nurse and student. Many staff nurses report that they find working with students challenging in that students raise questions and force the staff nurses to provide rationale for what they are doing.

Willingness to look at one's methods and rationale demonstrates both maturity and an interest in teaching and/or learning. Such role modeling by staff nurses is positive for students as it allows the student to observe mature, assertive behavior in responding to a criticism/critique. In addition, it reinforces to the student that a difference in opinion can be positive.

Resolution

The nurse in this situation did discuss her feelings with Joyce regarding the dressing change and was able to support her concerns with solid rationale. Joyce's response was unexpected. Joyce listened to the nurse's concerns and said she felt comfortable having the protocol changed. She said she had learned the same principles of microorganism transfer, but found that adhering to the principles "took too long."

Joyce agreed to reconsider her technique and to make another joint visit with the nurse the following day.

References

Baer, J. (1976). *How to be an assertive (not aggressive) woman, in life, in love and on the job.* New York: Signet.

Feeley, E. M., Shine, M. S., & Sloboda, S. B. (1980). *Fundamentals of nursing care.* New York: Van Nostrand.

Leslie, R. M., & Pakatar, C. S. (1980). Asepsis. In A. B. Saperstein & M. A. Frazier (Eds.). *Introduction to nursing practice.* Philadelphia: Davis (pp. 515–543).

Murray, B. S., & Valentine, A. S. (1981). *Intro-duction to nursing skills.* Burlington, VT: IDC Publications, University of Vermont.

Pointer, P., & Lancaster, J. (1984). Assertiveness in community health nursing. In M. Stanhope & J. Lancaster (Eds.). *Community health nursing.* St. Louis: Mosby (pp. 824–842).

Wykle, M. (1983). Adaptive behavior. In W. J. Phipps, B. C. Long, & N. F. Woods (Eds.). *Medical-surgical nursing.* (2d ed.) St. Louis: Mosby (pp. 177–201).

SITUATION 3
Mrs. Black: A Home Health Care Nursing Challenge (Self-Paced)

SECTION 3.1

Today is Tuesday. It is late afternoon and you have one more visit to make. Mrs. Black is a 65-year-old woman with several long-term problems. Her problem list reads as follows:

1. Diabetes mellitus (insulin dependent)
2. Atherosclerotic heart disease
   a. Angina 1976
   b. S/P MI 1977
   c. S/P pacemaker 1980
   d. CHF 1981
3. Bilateral cataracts

Mrs. Black's medications are:

Digoxin 0.25 mg p.o. qd
Lasix 40 mg p.o. bid
K-Ceil 20 mg p.o. bid (powder)
Nitroglycerin gr 1/150 S/L prn
   for chest pain

NPH insulin 25U s/c
Regular insulin 10U s/c $\Big\rangle$ 7 a.m.

NPH insulin 5U s/c
Regular insulin 5U s/c $\Big\rangle$ 5 p.m.

You see Mrs. Black every two weeks to monitor both her cardiac status and her diabetes. You have done much teaching with Mrs. Black and her family regarding medications, diet, and level of activity. Your visit today will focus on two areas:

1. Monitoring her cardiac status.
2. Observing the insulin preparation and administration.

Table 1 (next page) is a *cardiac flow sheet* for recording data when assessing Mrs. Black's cardiac status.

In the work space provided:

a. Indicate whether you think the list of parameters on the flow sheet is complete enough to assess Mrs. Black's cardiac status effectively. Write rationale for your decision.
   If you think the list is complete, stop here and proceed to page 28.
   If you think the list is incomplete . . .
b. *Add parameters to the flow sheet* which you think need to be included and note reason for additions.
c. List the questions or statements you will use to assess the parameters you have added.

Table 1. A Cardiac Flow Sheet

Parameters	Visit #1	Visit #2	Parameters	Visit #1	Visit #2
B/P					
Pulse: apical radial					
Rhythm: apical radial					
Heart sounds					
aortic					
pulmonic					
Erb's point					
tricuspid					
mitral					
Respirations					
quality					
breath sounds					
a) right					
b) left					
Extremities					
a) pulses					
b) color					
Edema (lower extremities)					
a) right					
b) left					
Neck veins					
Sensorium					
Ascites					
Weight					

Special Notations:

Student Work Space

Turn to the following pages to compare your answers.
a. enough parameters? – p. 28
b. additional parameters – p. 28
c. questions – p. 28

As you gather and record information, your flow sheet looks like Table 2, page 24.

SECTION 3.2

Based upon Mrs. Black's past medical history of a myocardial infarction and, more recently, congestive heart failure, it is also appropriate to assess her respiratory status. A change in cardiac status can have a direct effect upon her respiratory status.

In the work space provided:

a. Briefly describe how you would carry out a comprehensive respiratory assessment on Mrs. Black

Student Work Space

Turn to the following page to compare your answer.
a. respiratory assessment – p. 30

Table 2. A Completed Cardiac Flow Sheet

Parameters	Last Visit	Today's Visit
B/P	128/60	118/62
Pulse: apical	72	86
radial	72	86
Rhythm: apical	Regular	Regular
radial	Regular	Regular
Heart sounds		
aortic	Normal	Normal
pulmonic	Normal	Normal
Erb's point	Normal	Normal
tricuspid	Normal	Normal
mitral	Normal	Normal
Respirations	20	24
quality	even	slightly labored
breath sounds		
a) right	clear / clear	clear / fine rales (base)
b) left	clear / clear	clear / fine rales (base)
Extremities		
a) pulses	+/4 (strong)	+/4 (weak)
b) color	good	good
Edema (lower extremities)		
a) right	25 cm.	26.5 cm.
b) left	25 cm.	26.5 cm.
Neck veins	flat	slightly distended
Sensorium	alert oriented	alert oriented
Ascites	34"	34½"
Weight	148 lb	156 lb

Parameters	Last Visit	Today's Visit
Pain	denies	yes x2
location	–	substernal
duration		15 min each
severity		
frequency		x2
rel. to activity		when climbing stairs
Pain relief		yes with nitro gr 1/150
Palpitations	denies	denies
Fatigue/ Activity	takes a nap every p.m.	takes a nap every p.m.
Shortness of breath	denies	denies
Dyspnea	denies	when climbing stairs
Orthopnea	denies	denies
Syncope	denies	denies
Cough	yes / dry	yes / dry
Sputum	none	none
amount	–	–
color	–	–
consistency	–	–
Intake	2000 cc	2000 cc
Output	urine pale yellow	urine more concentrated
Diaphoresis	denies	denies

Special Notations:

Last Visit - RE: Respiratory Status
Fremitus: Equal bilaterally
Palpation: Equal bilaterally

Today's Visit - RE: Respiratory Status
Fremitus: Increased slightly at bases
Palpation: Equal bilaterally

SECTION 3.3 ————————————————

In your review of medications, Mrs. Black tells you that she is taking her medications "as usual." You ask her to identify each medication bottle and how she takes the medication.

Mrs. Black responds with the following:

> "My nitroglycerin gr 1/150 I take only if I have pain.
> Digoxin 0.25 mg, I take one at breakfast.
> Lasix 40 mg, I take one at breakfast and
> Potassium 20 mg, I take 1 packet of powder at breakfast and
>   supper.
> And of course my insulin, NPH 25U – regular 10U in the
>   morning and NPH 5U – regular 5U in the afternoon."

Based upon the information you have obtained from today's visit and recorded on the flow sheet, answer the following questions in the work space provided:

- a. State what you think about the information gathered on today's visit as compared to the same information gathered on the last visit.
- b. Is nursing intervention by you necessary? State your rationale.
  If no, stop here and proceed to page 36.
  If yes, describe your nursing intervention.
- c. Outline content for teaching you think is appropriate at this time for Mrs. Black. Support your teaching with rationale.

Student Work Space ——————————————————

Turn to the following pages to compare your answers.
a. information compared – p. 35
b. intervention? – p. 36
c. outline teaching – p. 37

SECTION 3.4

To complete your visit, you remind Mrs. Black that you want to observe her insulin preparation and injection technique. Mrs. Black is able to administer her insulin. However, because of her diminishing eyesight, she is not able to prepare it. Mrs. Black's 17-year-old granddaughter, Peggy, lives next door and has been preparing the injections (both insulins in one syringe). Peggy arrives to prepare her grandmother's insulin and she is aware you will be observing her. Peggy proceeds with the insulin preparation as follows:

1. Peggy opens a packet containing a new insulin syringe. She places the sterile syringe and an alcohol swab on the table. She takes a vial of U-100 regular insulin (clear) and a vial of U-100 NPH insulin (cloudy) from the refrigerator and places them on the table. (See Figure 2a.)
2. She washes her hands thoroughly and dries them.
3. She gently rotates the vial of NPH insulin in her hand.
4. She takes the alcohol swab and wipes the rubber stopper on both vials of insulin.
5. She removes the cap covering the needle of the syringe.
6. She inserts the needle of the syringe into the vial of NPH insulin, inverts the vial, draws up 5U of insulin, and removes the needle of the syringe from the vial. (See Figure 2b.)
7. She inserts the needle of the syringe into the vial of regular insulin, inverts the vial, draws up 5U of NPH insulin and removes the needle of the syringe from the vial.
8. She replaces the cap on the needle and hands the syringe to Mrs. Black.

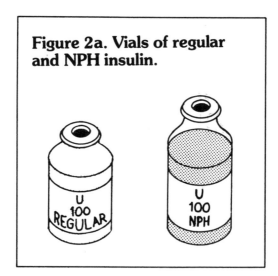

Figure 2a. Vials of regular and NPH insulin.

In the work space provided:

a. State whether or not you agree with Peggy's technique. Support your assessment with rationale.
b. What would your *initial response* be to Peggy's demonstration? Write your exact words.
c. If you agree with Peggy's technique, you may stop here.
   If you disagree with Peggy's technique, state how you would suggest she change it.

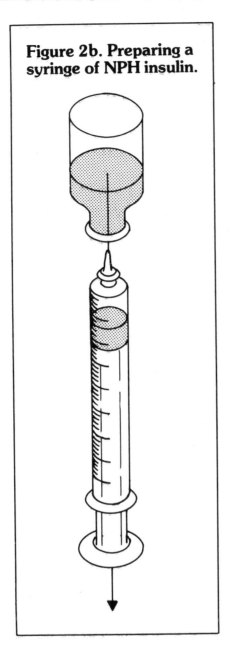

Figure 2b. Preparing a syringe of NPH insulin.

Student Work Space

Turn to the following pages to compare your answers.
a. agree/disagree with technique – p. 38
b. response to demonstration – p. 38
c. suggestion for change – p. 39

ANSWERS TO SECTION 3.1

a. Is the list of parameters complete enough to assess Mrs. Black's cardiac status effectively?

If you said the list of parameters is *not complete enough* to assess Mrs. Black's cardiac status effectively, *you are correct*. Although the parameters listed are all appropriate, they are all objective. There are no subjective parameters which together with the objective data would give a clearer impression of Mrs. Black's status. Subjective parameters serve as guidelines for soliciting relevant information from the client.

It is easy to become intrigued solely with the objective data collected, particularly as high technology has an increasing impact upon home health care and as nurses are expected to be more proficient in physical assessment. However, the most effective means of assessing a client is through the objective data in concert with the subjective data the client contributes (Dery, 1983).

b. Add parameters to the flow sheet that you think need to be included.

Compare the parameters you added to the flow sheet with the following list. If the majority of those you identified are listed here, congratulations!

Subjective parameters:

1. Pain
    a. location
    b. duration
    c. severity
    d. frequency
    e. relationship to activity
2. Pain relief
3. Palpitations
4. Fatigue/Activity
5. Shortness of breath
6. Dyspnea on exertion
7. Orthopnea
8. Syncope
9. Cough
10. Sputum
    a. amount
    b. color
    c. consistency
11. Fluid intake
12. Output
13. Diaphoresis
14. Edema

c. List the questions or statements you will use to assess the added parameters.

If the questions or statements you have identified are similar to those listed below, you are doing very well! Remember, when eliciting a history from a client, both questions and statements can be used. When possible, avoid using questions that imply the correct answer or closed-ended questions that may elicit only a "yes" or a "no." The more complete the information elicited from the client, the more accurate the assessment will be.

Parameters	Questions/statements
1. *Pain*	1. "Have you experienced any chest pain since my last visit?"
a. *location*	"Please describe the pain you experienced; show me where it occurred;
b. *duration*	describe how it felt in your own words;
c. *severity*	estimate how long it lasted each time;
d. *frequency*	describe what you were doing when it
e. *relationship to activity*	occurred."
	If she denies pain, rephrase the question, eliminating the word "pain" and substituting words such as "pressure,"

"squeezing," "knifelike," "discomfort," "heartburn," "discomfort in arm, neck, or jaw," all of which are common manifestations of cardiac pain.

Another means of rephrasing would be to ask her if she has taken any nitroglycerin since your last visit. If she admits to any of the above, then ask her to describe the feeling, show you exactly where it occurred, describe how it felt (intensity), and estimate how long it lasted.

2. *Pain relief*

2. "Tell me what you did to relieve the 'pain,' 'discomfort,' etc.," is better than "Did you take the nitroglycerin?" Here you are looking for use of medication, i.e., nitroglycerin, change of position, use of oxygen, or a home remedy.

3. *Palpitations* (Kavanagh & Riegger, 1983; Malasanos et al., 1985)

3. "Have you experienced palpitations (a pounding sensation) in your chest?" "Has your heart felt as though it was racing?"

4. *Fatigue/Activity* (Kavanagh & Riegger, 1983)

4. "Please tell me about your physical activity since my last visit."

5. *Shortness of breath*

5. "Have you noticed any changes in your breathing since my last visit?"

6. *Dyspnea* (Kavanagh & Riegger, 1983; Malasanos, Barkauskas, Moss, & Stoltenberg-Allen, 1985; Baldwin, 1983)

6. This is an area where the initial question may need to be rephrased, e.g., "Does climbing stairs affect your breathing?"

7. *Orthopnea* (Kavanagh & Riegger, 1983; Malasanos et al., 1985; Baldwin, 1983)

7. "How many pillows are you using when you sleep?"

8. *Syncope* (Kavanagh & Riegger, 1983; Malasanos et al., 1985; Baldwin, 1983)

8. "Have you experienced lightheadedness or generalized weakness on bending over or standing upright?" "Please describe how you felt."

9. *Cough* (Malasanos et al., 1985)

9. "Have you experienced a cough since my last visit?" "What time of day does it occur?" "Are you coughing up any sputum?"

10. *Sputum* (Malasanos et al., 1985)

10. If yes, "Please describe the color, consistency, and amount of sputum."

(continued)

Parameters	*Questions/statements*
11. *Intake*	11. "Tell me how much fluid you have been drinking in a 24-hour period." May need to go through day meal by meal including snacks to obtain accurate data. Be certain to ascertain the size of the cup or glass used.
12. *Output*	12. "Please describe the color of your urine." "Have you noticed any change in the amount of urine you are passing in a 24-hour period?" "Please describe." Be sure to inquire about changes, especially frequency or nocturia.
13. *Diaphoresis*	13. "Have you noticed any change in the amount of perspiration?" "Please describe."
14. *Edema* (Kavanagh & Riegger, 1983; Malasanos et al., 1985)	14. "Have you experienced any swelling in your feet or hands?" "Do your shoes fit more tightly at night than in the morning?"

ANSWERS TO SECTION 3.2

a. Briefly describe how you would carry out a comprehensive respiratory assessment on Mrs. Black.

With more and more patients being discharged from hospitals early, or not being admitted to hospitals at all, refined physical assessment skills have become an integral part of the home health nurse's practice whether the client has a long-term chronic illness or an acute illness. With the physical assessment skills comes the responsibility to perform the skills correctly. Obviously, assessment skills performed incorrectly will result in inaccurate data collection, inaccurate assessments, and inappropriate or inadequate care.

Nurses are increasingly assuming responsibility for assessing respiratory function. The following description of a respiratory assessment would be appropriate to use with Mrs. Black. The four components of physical assessment will be addressed; inspection, palpation, percussion, and auscultation.

If your description of a comprehensive respiratory assessment resembles this one, you have a good knowledge base. If it does not, take time to identify the areas of difference. To gain more confidence and skill in physical assessment the following are suggested:

1. *Read* on the techniques of physical assessment.
2. *View* films on physical assessment and listen to audio tapes, i.e., breath sounds, heart sounds, in your audiovisual library.
3. *Ask* your clinical instructor for guidance in the skills laboratory and the clinical setting.
4. *PRACTICE* your skills on healthy adults and children. There is a wide variation in normal. Having an accurate perception of normal makes identifying abnormal sounds less difficult.
5. Most of all, *THINK* about the assessment process, the data you're gathering, what it means, *and* how the data fit with what the client is saying.

Respiratory Assessment. Perform respiratory assessment in the following sequence:

1. Select a warm, private, well-lighted area for the physical assessment.
2. Ask the client to assume an unsupported sitting position.
3. Have the client remove all clothing from the waist up; the presence of clothing on the chest wall can alter the sounds elicited.

Inspection. Observe the client for the following:

1. Skin
    a. Rashes – type, color, location
    b. Scars – resulting from surgery or trauma
2. Size and symmetry of chest – i.e., barrel-shaped, kyphosis, lordosis, scoliosis
3. Breathing pattern
    a. Rate
    b. Rhythm
    c. Depth
    d. Thoracic expansion – is it symmetrical? To observe thoracic expansion, place your thumbs at the level of the client's tenth ribs and extend the palms of your hands on the posteriolateral chest wall. You will be able to feel the chest wall expand (Malasanos et al., 1985; Wyper, Daly, & Norman, 1983).

Palpation. Palpate for tactile fremitus as follows:

1. Place the palmar bases of your fingers on the client's posterior chest beginning at the shoulders.
2. Ask the client to repeat "ninety-nine" or "one-one-one" and feel the vibration in your hands; compare the vibrations felt.
3. Move both hands down the chest wall, simultaneously, to below the scapula and then below the diaphragm. In each of these places, feel the vibrations as the client again says "ninety-nine" (Malasanos et al., 1985; Wyper et al., 1983).
4. The anterior and lateral chest are examined in this fashion. Tactile fremitus is normal and is present in the healthy adult. The fremitus should be equal side to side (slight variations are normal) beginning as a soft buzzing in the upper lobes to almost nothing in the lower lobes. Fremitus may be difficult to feel in a client with a soft or high-pitched voice. This can be remedied by asking the client to lower the tone of voice.

    Increased fremitus may occur when a consolidation occurs within the lung tissue, i.e., pneumonia, tumor, pulmonary fibrosis (Malasanos et al., 1985, p. 300). Decreased or absent fremitus occurs when sounds are decreased or when sounds must pass through added medium, i.e., pleural effusion, pleural thickening, pneumothorax, bronchial obstruction, or emphysema (Malasanos et al., 1985, p. 300).

Percussion. Percuss the chest as follows (if you are right-handed):

1. Place the palmar surface of the fingers on your left hand on the posterior chest wall.
2. Place the middle finger in an intercostal space between two ribs.
3. Exert a slightly harder pressure on the chest wall with the middle finger.
4. With the end of the middle finger of the right hand, tap sharply on the middle phalanx of the middle finger on the left hand. The tapping

action should come from the wrist, not the elbow or the shoulder (Malasanos et al., 1985; Wyper et al., 1983).

Percussion should be done on the posterior and anterior chest in the areas and sequence identified in the illustrations which follow. (See Figures 3 and 4.) Move side to side comparing the sounds elicited. The lateral chest walls should be percussed.

The following sounds can be elicited through percussion:

1. Resonance – an echoing sound produced when air is present. Resonance is elicited when the chest of a healthy adult is percussed.
2. Hyperresonance – sounds a little more drumlike as more than the normal amount of air is trapped in the lung, as with the asthmatic or emphysemic client.
3. Tympany – sounds like a kettledrum; occurs when there is air in the pleural cavity, as in pneumothorax.
4. Dullness – sounds like a thud; occurs when there is a consolidation of some type within the lung, as in pneumonia or a tumor. (Some dullness will be elicited on the anterior chest over the heart and liver.)

Auscultation. Auscultate the posterior and anterior chest as follows:

1. Ask the client to breathe through the mouth and slightly deeper than usual to make the breath sounds more audible.
2. Keep the tubing of your stethoscope from rubbing against the client's chest or your clothing to avoid creating extraneous sounds.
3. Place the diaphragm of your stethoscope firmly against the client's chest during auscultation. Auscultation should be done on the posterior and anterior chest in the areas and sequence identified in the illustrations which follow. (See Figures 5 and 6.) Some nurses elect, with elderly clients, to begin auscultation at the bases and work upward toward the shoulders. This allows the nurse to hear the softer sounds at the bases before the client tires.

The following are normal breath sounds (Malasanos et al., 1985; Wyper et al., 1983):

Bronchial(tubular/tracheal) – all of inspiration and expiration is heard. These sounds are normal when heard over the trachea. They are abnormal when heard over the peripheral lung.
Vesicular – normal breath sounds. All of inspiration is heard and very little of expiration is heard. These sounds resemble a soft breeze blowing through the trees.
Bronchovesicular – all of inspiration and some of expiration is heard. These sounds are normal when heard in areas of the major bronchi, especially in the area of the right lung and at the sternal borders.

The following are abnormal breath sounds or adventitious sounds (Malasanos et al., 1985; Wyper et al., 1983):

Rales – short, discrete, interrupted crackling sounds most commonly heard on inspiration.
Fine rales – high-pitched sounds similar to those you can produce by rubbing strands of hair between your fingers in front of your ear. Occurring later in inspiration, they are often heard at the bases with congestive heart failure.
Medium rales – medium-pitched, louder than fine rales. Heard mid-inspiration.

Figure 3. Appropriate sequence for percussion of the posterior chest.

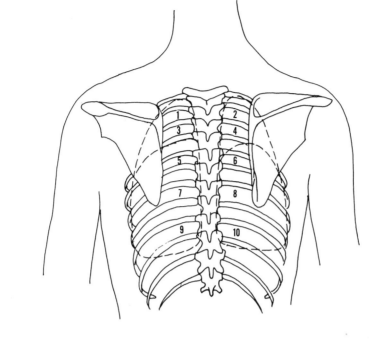

Figure 4. Appropriate sequence for percussion of the anterior chest.

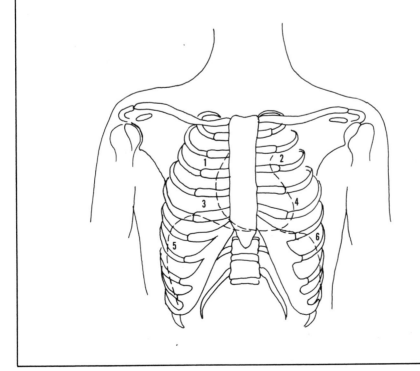

Figure 5. Appropriate sequence for auscultation of the posterior chest.

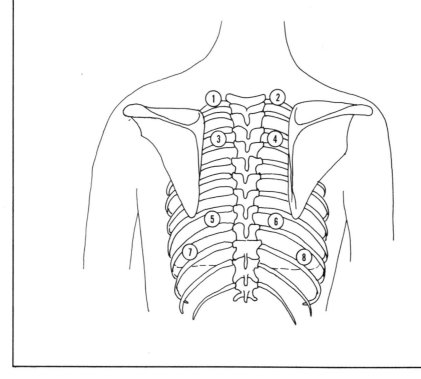

Figure 6. Appropriate sequence for auscultation of the anterior chest.

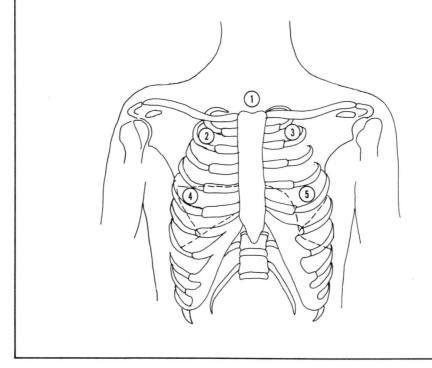

Coarse rales – low-pitched, similar to the crackling of a fire. They are louder than medium and fine rales. They occur early in inspiration and are thought to have their origin in the bronchi.

Rhonchi – continuous sounds produced by the movement of air through passages of the tracheobronchial tree which have been narrowed by secretions, swelling, or tumors.

Sibilant – continuous high-pitched, wheezing sounds; may be heard on inspiration and expiration but predominantly on expiration.

Sonorous – continuous, low-pitched, moaning or snoring sounds. They may be heard on inspiration and expiration but predominantly on expiration.

Friction rub – a creaking or grating sound caused by the rubbing together of inflamed and roughened pleural surfaces. Heard on both inspiration and expiration in the lower anterolateral chest.

ANSWERS TO SECTION 3.3

a. What do you conclude from the data gathered on today's visit as compared to the same data gathered on the last visit?

If you stated that *the changes* in Mrs. Black's objective and subjective parameters *are significant* and need to be addressed, *you are correct.*

The following parameters are those in which you should have noted changes:

1. Blood pressure – decreased systolic; slightly increased diastolic
2. Pulse – both apical and radial are increased
3. Respirations – increased
4. Quality of respirations – have become slightly labored
5. Chest sounds – fine basilar rales have appeared
   Special notations: fremitus is increased slightly in the same area that the rales are heard
6. Extremities – pulses are weaker
7. Ankle edema – increased 1½ cm
8. Neck veins – slightly distended
9. Ascites – increased ½ in.
10. Weight – increased 8 lb
11. Pain – she admits to two episodes of substernal pain lasting 15 minutes; both episodes associated with activity; both relieved with nitroglycerin
12. Dyspnea – has noticed when climbing stairs
13. Fluid intake and output – intake has remained consistent while output has decreased

Based upon these changes, it looks as though the level of Mrs. Black's cardiac decompensation is increasing. She seems to be demonstrating some symptoms associated with both right-sided and left-sided failure.

Right-sided failure – right ventricle hypertrophies because of increased pressure in pulmonary artery; blood not effectively moved into the lungs for aeration. Blood backs up in superior and inferior vena cava, causing a pitting-type edema in extremities. Neck veins become distended (Kavanagh, 1983).

Left-sided failure – weakened left ventricle cannot effectively pump oxygenated blood into arterial circulation. Ineffective pumping causes blood to back up in pulmonary vessels producing pulmonary congestion and edema. Labored breathing and shortness of breath occur (Kavanagh, 1983).

In addition, *if you identified the error in* Mrs. Black's *medication regimen, you are sharp!* Mrs. Black identified each of her medications correctly. However, when describing how she takes them, she indicated that she took her Lasix 40 mg once a day, at breakfast; the information you have indicates that Lasix 40 mg p.o. was ordered to be taken twice a day. This error in the medication regimen could be a factor in Mrs. Black's increased cardiac decompensation.

Medication errors in the elderly population are common. Some of the problems are outdated drugs, taking prn drugs too often, visual impairment, childproof containers, and omission of regularly scheduled doses (Mullen & Granholm, 1981).

If you stated that *the changes* in Mrs. Black's objective and subjective parameters *are not significant* and do not need to be addressed, your answer is *incorrect.*

Your rationale may have been that the changes do not seem major and perhaps could be reassessed in a day or two. In some situations, where there are a few small changes, this might be true. In this situation, however, there are many changes in the objective parameters as well as in the subjective information given by Mrs. Black. A change in status can occur very quickly in long-term cardiac clients; what may seem like small changes should not be overlooked.

In addition to the changes, there is an error in the way Mrs. Black is taking her medications, an error that could be contributing to the changes in her cardiac status. Read the above correct answer.

b. Is nursing intervention necessary? What will you do?

Yes, nursing intervention is necessary. The changes in the objective and subjective parameters are significant and the error in medication is significant. As a skilled professional it is your responsibility to intervene. The following actions would be appropriate:

1. Ask the client if her physician told her to change the dosage of her Lasix.
2. Explain to the client that you have found some changes in her status during this visit, i.e., increased pulse, increased respirations, increased edema, fine rales, error in medication, and that in light of these changes intervention is needed. (Be careful not to frighten the client when presenting this information.)
3. *Notify physician* with data collected comparing data from today's visit with data from the previous visit. When presenting your data be clear and concise. Present data in a logical order, i.e., all objective data with changes and all subjective data with changes. It will be at the discretion of the individual nurse whether notification of the physician occurs during the visit or at the conclusion of the visit. Attempt to contact physician from client's home. If physician is not available, leave message with secretary adding you will call again. Advise client of situation and tell her you will call her after talking with her physician.
4. Be prepared to take verbal orders for medication changes. In community settings it is not only appropriate but essential to take verbal orders. If the nurse were required to wait for written orders to arrive by mail, the client's care could be compromised. Driving to a physician's office to have orders signed is not an efficient use of the nurse's time. The above refers only to community settings where a physician is not on site. *The practice of not taking verbal orders in a hospital setting is still maintained.* Verbal orders will need to be validated on

whatever form the home health agency/VNA uses for documenting orders. The form is then sent to the physician for a signature. If you, as a student, are completing such a form for validation of verbal orders, have it countersigned by a staff nurse or nursing supervisor before sending it to the physician.

5. Clarify medication changes with the physician by reading the changed orders you've noted back over the phone. The physician may want to restart Lasix as ordered (bid) or increase the dosage substantially for one or two days.
6. Clarify the orders from the physician with the client.

c. **Outline content for teaching and support with rationale.**

Teaching	*Rationale*
1. Clarify medication changes with client/family.	1. Avoid further medication errors.
2. Review how and when to use the nitroglycerin. Check age of nitroglycerin; suggest fresh supply if older than 3-6 months.	2. Reassure the client that use of the nitroglycerin is appropriate. Help client to reinforce differences between musculoskeletal pain and angina (Pinneo, 1984). Nitroglycerin deteriorates and loses strength with age once the bottle is opened.
3. Pathophysiology surrounding the changes	3. A succinct, uncomplicated explanation may help the client to understand why she has experienced the recent changes.
4. Elevation of lower extremities and use of elastic stockings	4. Increase venous return; decrease edema by decreasing pooling in dependent extremities (Kavanagh, 1983; Brunner & Suddarth, 1984).
5. Physical activity	5. Discuss ways to avoid overexertion, i.e., climbing stairs, lifting, which result in increased cardiac workload.
6. Balanced periods of rest/exercise	6. Avoid overexertion and increased cardiac workload (Kavanagh, 1983; Brunner & Suddarth, 1984).
7. Small, frequent meals	7. Decrease cardiac workload (Kavanagh, 1983; Brunner & Suddarth, 1984).
8. Sodium intake	8. If client is on a sodium-restricted diet, review foods naturally high in sodium and those to which sodium is added, i.e., pickles, catsup, etc. Increased fluid retention leads to increased cardiac workload (Kavanagh, 1983; Brunner & Suddarth, 1984).
9. Skin care	9. Maintain skin integrity of edematous extremities; edematous extremities are poorly nourished and are susceptible to breakdown (Kavanagh, 1983).

ANSWERS TO SECTION 3.4

a. Do you agree/disagree with Peggy's technique? State your rationale.

If you disagreed with Peggy's technique, *you are correct.* Peggy does a pretty good job in preparing Mrs. Black's insulin with two exceptions:

1. Air was not injected into each vial before drawing up the insulin; if this is done repeatedly, a vacuum will form inside the vial and the first dose of insulin in the syringe could easily be pulled into the second vial.
2. The NPH insulin was drawn up before the regular insulin; when a long-acting insulin and regular insulin are mixed in the same syringe, the regular insulin is drawn up first to prevent the possibility of any long-acting insulin getting into the vial of regular insulin. If such contamination does occur, it is preferable and safer to have a minute amount of the regular insulin added to the NPH than the long-acting NPH added to the regular insulin.

b. What would your initial response be to Peggy's demonstration? Write your exact words.

Your initial response to Peggy's demonstration needs to be one that will facilitate effective communication between you and Peggy as well as encourage her continued participation in her grandmother's care. Your initial response needs to convey the following:

- *acknowledgment* of Peggy's participation
- *respect* for Peggy as an individual
- *identification* of areas of strength in the technique
- *identification* of areas for improvement and rationale
- *reassurance* that you will help her with the areas that need improvement

Here are some examples to compare with your initial response:

"Thank you for demonstrating for me. I can see that you understand the importance of hand washing, gentle rotation of the NPH insulin, and maintaining sterility and accuracy of the doses. I did notice two areas that can be improved. Those are . . . Let me show you and explain why as well as answer any questions you may have."

"I appreciate your taking the time to demonstrate for me. I think your technique has some strong points, such as . . . There are also two areas which I would encourage you to change. Those are . . . I can demonstrate and I'll be happy to answer any questions."

Notice the use of the "I" statements in the above examples. Use of the "I" statement is beneficial in maintaining clear communication. By beginning the statement with "I," the speaker is assuming all responsibility for what is about to be said. Generally, people respond positively to "I" statements, and their positive response allows them to hear the total statement. In learning communication skills as children, many of us are not taught to use the "I" statement effectively. Instead we are taught to use the ineffective "You" statement. "You did this . . ." "Why didn't you do that?" "You" statements are accusatory in nature and make the person receiving them feel uncomfortable, perhaps defensive, and even angry (Pointer & Lancaster, 1984).

Look at your initial response. Are there "I" statements or are there "You" statements which may be perceived by Peggy as negative or accusatory and could result in anger or defensiveness? Statements producing these results with Peggy would be inappropriate.

c. How would you suggest Peggy change her technique?

The following technique would be appropriate for Peggy to use when preparing two types of insulin in one syringe.

1. Wash hands thoroughly (Leslie & Pakatar, 1980; Murray & Valentine, 1981).
2. Gather equipment.
3. Gently rotate the vial of NPH insulin to mix the suspension uniformly through the solution (Sims, 1980).
4. Cleanse the rubber stopper in both vials with an alcohol swab and friction.
5. Into the vial of NPH insulin (cloudy), inject 5U of air. For displacement, the amount of air injected is equal to the amount of insulin to be removed. Remove the syringe from the vial *without* drawing up the insulin.
6. Into the vial of regular insulin (clear), inject 5U of air for displacement. Invert the vial and draw up 5U regular into the syringe; observe closely for air bubbles; remove the needle from the vial.
7. Reinsert the needle of the syringe into the vial of NPH insulin (cloudy) and draw up 5U of NPH insulin, being careful not to allow any regular insulin to leak into the NPH vial; observe closely for air bubbles; remove the needle of the syringe from the vial.
8. Replace the cap on the needle of the syringe (Sims, 1980).

Resolution

Peggy was not defensive when approached by the nurse. She asked several questions regarding the order of the insulin withdrawal and said she was relieved to know that now she really understood what she was doing and why.

Mrs. Black's injection technique was observed and positive reinforcement given for her technique.

Near the conclusion of the visit, Mrs. Black's doctor was notified regarding the numerous changes in her parameters and the error in the medication regimen. The physician ordered Mrs. Black's Lasix dosage to be increased to 40 mg *tid* for two days; then returning to bid order. The nurse carefully explained and wrote down the doctor's orders for Mrs. Black, helping her to plan when she could conveniently take the third dose of Lasix for the next two days. She felt confident that Mrs. Black understood when to return to the bid dosage and planned a revisit in a week. On returning to the office, the nurse initiated the process to obtain a written confirmation of the order change from the physician.

When the nurse visited Mrs. Black the following week, she found that Mrs. Black's symptoms had resolved, she was following the correct medication regimen, and she was feeling better.

References

Baldwin, P. J. (1983). Nursing care of the elderly person with an acute cardiovascular problem. *Nursing Clinics of North America* 18(2):385–394.

Brunner, L. S., & Suddarth, D. S. (1984). *Textbook of medical-surgical nursing.* New York: Lippincott.

Dery, G. K. (1983). The problem-oriented system. In W. J. Phipps, B. C. Long, & N. F. Woods (Eds.). *Medical-surgical nursing.* (2d ed.) St. Louis: Mosby (pp. 130–145).

Kavanagh, J. M. (1983). Problems of the heart and major blood vessels. In W. J. Phipps, B. C. Long, & N. F. Woods (Eds.). *Medical-surgical nursing.* (2d ed.) St. Louis: Mosby (pp. 1099–1141).

Kavanagh, J. M., & Riegger, M. J. (1983). Assessment of the cardiovascular system and intervention for the person with a cardiovascular problem. In W. J. Phipps, B. C. Long, & N. F. Woods (Eds.). *Medical-surgical nursing.* (2d ed.) St. Louis: Mosby (pp. 1029–1064; 1065–1098).

Leslie, R. M., & Pakatar, C. S. (1980). Asepsis. In A. B. Saperstein & M. A. Frazier (Eds.). *Introduction to nursing practice.* Philadelphia: Davis (pp. 515–543).

Malasanos, L., Barkauskas, V., Moss, M., & Stoltenberg-Allen, K. (1985). *Health assessment.* St. Louis: Mosby.

Mullen, E., & Granholm, M. (1981). Drugs and the elderly patient. *Journal of Gerontological Nursing* 7(2):108–113.

Murray, B. S., & Valentine, A. S. (1981). *Introduction to nursing skills.* Burlington, VT: IDC Publications, University of Vermont.

Pinneo, R. (1984). Living with coronary artery disease. *Nursing Clinics of North America* 19(3):459–467.

Pointer, P., & Lancaster, J. (1984). Assertiveness in community health nursing. In M. Stanhope & J. Lancaster (Eds.). *Community health nursing.* St. Louis: Mosby (pp. 824–842).

Sims, D. (1980). *Diabetes: Reach for health and freedom.* St. Louis: Mosby.

Wyper, M. A., Daly, B. J., & Norman, A. (1983). Assessment of the respiratory system. In W. J. Phipps, B. C. Long, & N. F. Woods (Eds.). *Medical-surgical nursing.* (2d ed.) St. Louis: Mosby (pp. 1212–1225).

∿∿∿∿∿ SITUATION 4 ∿∿∿∿∿
Setting Priorities:
Managing a Caseload
∿∿∿∿ (Group Discussion) ∿∿∿∿

SECTION 4.1 ─────────────────────

Today is Monday. Upon your arrival at the home health agency your supervisor tells you that the continuing care coordinator at the local hospital has called and requested the presence of a community health nurse (CHN) at a discharge planning conference; both clients will be assigned to your caseload. Since the conference will be held this afternoon, you will be able to visit only four clients instead of the six you have scheduled.

Review the list of clients given in Table 3 (next page), and in the work space provided below determine the following:

- a. The four clients you will visit today.
- b. The order in which you will visit them.
- c. Your rationale for visiting in the order you've identified.
- d. How will you reschedule the clients you are not going to visit today?

Student Work Space ─────────────────────────────

41

Table 3. Clients to Visit

Client (Age)	Diagnosis	Frequency of visits	Length of visits	Client history
Edward Grove (68)	S/P colostomy, chronic lung disease	Daily by CHN	1 hr	Client had a lengthy hospital admission with a variety of complications (has frequent URI's). Discharged prior to having full understanding of colostomy irrigation. CHN has done majority of teaching. Last seen on Friday; did his own irrigation alone for the first time Sat./Sun. (at his request). Lives alone.
Rachel Wind (70)	Chronic lung disease, ASHD with recurrent angina	Every two weeks by CHN. Mon. & Thurs. by HH aide	45 min-1 hr	CHN monitors cardiac and respiratory status. HH aide assists with personal care. Client generally has psychosocial problems she wants to discuss on each visit. Lives alone.
Robert Arthur (59)	S/P posterior MI, CHF	Twice a week by CHN	45 min	Last seen on Friday, at which time he showed evidence of +1 pitting edema bilaterally lower extremities (an increase from trace edema on previous visit). Visits from CHN have resulted in frequent medication adjustments via telephone from the physician. (Meds: Lasix, Hydralazine, Digoxin, and a potassium supplement.) He refuses further hospital admission. Lives with wife.

SECTION 4.2

New Information

To be read by faculty member.

Table 3 (continued)

Client (Age)	Diagnosis	Frequency of visits	Length of visits	Client history
Alfred Walsh (73)	Alzheimer's disease; reportedly abused by son	Monthly by CHN. Monthly by social worker. Daily by HH aide	45 min	Client has become increasingly confused during the past year; he can no longer provide his own personal care. Four months ago neighbors reported he was being physically abused by his son. CHN works closely with social workers in monitoring for abuse; also provides health care maintenance. HH aide provides personal care and observes for sign of abuse. Lives with son and his family.
Norma Turner (59)	Infected suture lines, S/P femoral/ popliteal bypass (done 2 months ago). Abdominal wound 2 by 2½ by 1 in.; R groin wound 2 by 1½ by ½ in.	Twice a week by CHN	1–1½ hr	Dressings are changed twice a day. Procedure includes (1) assist client with shower for debridement, (2) heat lamp for 20 minutes, (3) pack wounds and redress. Client is not on antibiotics. Client is frequently confused. She lives with and is cared for by her daughter.
Ellen Carter (45)	Paranoid schizophrenic	Every two weeks by CHN	30 min	CHN administers Prolixin injection every two weeks. Prolixin was due yesterday; must not be delayed over 24 hours from scheduled time. Client becomes extremely anxious at injection time. Lives with her mother.

Note: All clients have telephones; all live within one block of one another.

In the work space provided determine the following:

    a. Should this client be seen today?
    b. If no, why? If yes, state rationale and *reprioritize clients.*
    c. If yes, what will you be looking for?
    d. Identify the parameters you will use in your assessment.

Student Work Space

SECTION 4.3

Client to be seen first: Name: _____

Clinical Findings

To be read by faculty member.

In the work space provided:

    a. State your assessment.
    b. Based upon your assessment, what do you do?

Student Work Space

SECTION 4.4

Client to be seen second: Name: _____

> **New Information**
>
> To be read by faculty member.

In the work space provided:

  a. Identify the parameters you will monitor in assessing this client.

Student Work Space

SECTION 4.5

> **Clinical Findings**
>
> To be read by faculty member.

Based upon clinical findings, in the work space provided:

a. State your assessment, based upon rationale.
b. State plans based upon assessment and immediate action you will take.
c. When should this client be seen again?

Student Work Space

SECTION 4.6

Client to be seen third: Name: _____

> **Clinical Findings**
> To be read by faculty member.

In the work space provided:

    a. Do you feel this client's complaints are significant? Why?

    b. Do you have enough data to make an assessment? If yes, state your assessment and rationale. If no, determine what further data are needed.

Student Work Space

SECTION 4.7

Clinical Findings

To be read by faculty member.

In the work space provided:

a. State your assessment.
b. Based upon your assessment, what do you do?

Student Work Space

Suggested Reading

American Red Cross (1979). *Advanced first aid and emergency care.* (2d ed.) Garden City, NY: Doubleday.

Brunner, L. S., & Suddarth, D. S. (1984). *Textbook of medical-surgical nursing.* New York: Lippincott.

Cassmeyer, V. L., Mitten, C. J., & Phipps, W. J. (1983). Problems of the endocrine system. In W. J. Phipps, B. C. Long, & N. F. Woods (Eds.). *Medical-surgical nursing.* (2d ed.) St. Louis: Mosby (pp. 615–675).

Dery, G. K. (1983). The problem-oriented system. In W. J. Phipps, B. C. Long, & N. F. Woods (Eds.). *Medical-surgical nursing.* (2d ed.) St. Louis: Mosby (pp. 130–145).

Hahn, A. B., Barkin, R. L., & Oestreich, S. J. K. (1982). *Pharmacology in nursing.* (15th ed.) St. Louis: Mosby.

Kavanagh, J. M. (1983). Problems of the heart and major blood vessels. In W. J. Phipps, B. C. Long, & N. F. Woods (Eds.). *Medical-surgical nursing.* (2d ed.) St. Louis: Mosby (pp. 1099–1141).

Kavanagh, J. M., & Riegger, M. J. (1983). Assessment of the cardiovascular system and intervention for the person with a cardiovascular problem. In W. J. Phipps, B. C. Long, & N. F. Woods (Eds.). *Medical-surgical nursing.* (2d ed.) St. Louis: Mosby (pp. 1029–1064; 1065–1098).

Leslie, R. M., & Pakatar, C. S. (1980). Asepsis. In A. B. Saperstein & M. A. Frazier (Eds.). *Introduction to nursing practice.* Philadelphia: Davis (pp. 515–543).

Lockhart, C. (1979). Family-focused community health nursing services in the home. In S. E. Archer & R. P. Fleshman (Eds.). *Community health nursing.* (2d ed.) Belmont, CA: Wadsworth (pp. 152–175).

Malasanos, L., Barkauskas, V., Moss, M., & Stoltenberg-Allen, K. (1981). *Health assessment.* St. Louis: Mosby.

Murray, B. S., & Valentine, A. S. (1981). *Introduction to nursing skills.* Burlington, VT: IDC Publications, University of Vermont.

Soltis, B. (1983). Fluid and electrolyte imbalance. In W. J. Phipps, B. C. Long, & N. F. Woods (Eds.). *Medical-surgical nursing.* (2d ed.) St. Louis: Mosby (pp. 327–358).

Wyper, M. A., Daly, B. J., & Norman, A. (1983). Assessment of the respiratory system. In W. J. Phipps, B. C. Long, & N. F. Woods (Eds.). *Medical-surgical nursing.* (2d ed.) St. Louis: Mosby (pp. 1212–1225).

SITUATION 5
Middletown: A Community as Client (Self-Paced)

SECTION 5.1

You are the nursing supervisor at the Middletown Home Health Care Agency. This is a private, nonprofit agency that serves Middletown, a community of 15,000 near Boston. The agency has attempted to meet the needs of Middletown residents with the following programs:

Population	Services provided
a. Preschool children	Well-child clinics, including physical examinations, developmental assessments, immunizations, anticipatory guidance, and nutrition education for parents.
b. Maternal-child health	Prenatal classes; support groups for pregnant women; support groups for new mothers and families.
c. School-age children	Full-time school nursing services provided by a contractual agreement with the town in the three elementary schools and the high school; the nurses participate in providing health education to individuals and groups.
d. Middle adult	Home care for individuals with acute and chronic illnesses; family support; blood pressure screening and follow-up program.
e. Elderly	Home care for individuals with acute and chronic illnesses; blood pressure screening and follow-up; exercise and nutrition education programs; support groups for widows and widowers.

During the past year, the director of the agency has raised questions about the health care of the middle adult population of Middletown. Since there are only two physicians in the town and the nearest emergency room is over ten miles away, she thinks their needs are not adequately met.

As a solution, the director has proposed that agency's board of directors support the establishment of an ambulatory care facility staffed by nurse practitioners to meet the acute and chronic health care needs of Middletown's adult population. The board of directors is intrigued by the idea.

In the work space provided:

    a. State whether or not you think the board of directors should support the director's proposal. State your rationale.
    b. If yes, stop here.
       If no, describe how you think the board of directors should proceed.

Student Work Space

Turn to the following pages to compare your answers.
a. support/not support proposal – p. 59
b. how to proceed – p. 60

SECTION 5.2

You have been asked to work with another nurse over the next few months to complete a comprehensive community assessment and make recommendations to the board of directors based upon your findings. You agree to do so.

In thinking about the project you realize that before proceeding, the terms "community" and "community assessment" need to be clearly defined.

In the work space provided:

   a. Define community.
   b. Define community assessment.

Student Work Space

Turn to the following pages to compare your answers.
a. define community – p. 60
b. define community assessment – p. 62

SECTION 5.3

The initial phases of your community assessment focus on data gathering. As you begin, questions arise regarding what type of data should be gathered, what relevance the data have to the assessment, and where the data can be found. Listed below are nine major categories for which objective data can be gathered, and one category of subjective data.

In the work space provided:

   a. Describe the relevance of the data, in each of the ten major categories, to the community assessment.
   b. State where you think the data for each of the categories can be found.

Student Work Space

Community Assessment Data

Type	Relevance	Source of information
Objective data:		

1. *Your observations of the community*
  a. geographic boundaries
  b. housing quality
  c. neighborhood gathering places
  d. characteristics of street people
  e. readily observable qualities
  (Goeppinger, 1984)		

(continued)

Type	Relevance	Source of information
2. *Geographical description of the community*		
a. size, area		
b. topography, description of land		
c. location of community in terms of		
(1) natural resources		
(2) trade/travel routes		
(3) other communities		
d. terrain, access roads		
e. agricultural/ industrial		
f. residential		
g. climate		
h. environmental pollution		
(Klein, 1982; Spradley, 1985)		
3. *Descriptors of the population*		
a. population		
b. population growth/ shrinkage		
c. population projections		
d. racial/nationality makeup		
e. population by age breakdown		
f. education level		
g. average income		
h. range of income		
i. religion		
j. types of employment		
k. rate of employment		
(Spradley, 1985)		
l. rate of unemployment		
m. number on welfare		
n. rate of divorce		

Type	Relevance	Source of information
o. number of single-parent families		
p. crime rate (1) major crimes (2) juvenile delinquency (3) rate of DWI (Burgess, 1976)		
4. *Community services*		
a. fire protection		
b. police protection		
c. shopping facilities		
d. public transportation		
e. water supply		
f. sewage disposal		
5. *Community resources*		
a. day care centers		
b. schools/vocational programs/colleges		
c. parks, playgrounds/ recreational facilities (tennis courts, swimming pools)		
d. elderly housing		
6. *Health resources*		
a. hospitals		
b. emergency services		
c. physicians		
d. home health agency		
e. mental health programs		
f. self-help groups		
g. state health programs		
h. pharmacy		
i. nursing homes (Rodgers, 1984; Spradley, 1985)		

(continued)

Type	Relevance	Source of information
7. *Morbidity/mortality statistics* a. mortality rates —age adjusted b. infant mortality rate c. mortality rates by cause—age adjusted d. morbidity rate (Spradley, 1985) 8. *Community power structure* a. form of government b. community officials c. community members controlling: (1) industry (2) natural resources (3) financial reserves (Klein, 1982; Spradley, 1985) 9. *Community survey/questionnaire* Formal gathering of data from community residents to compare with the preceding information. a. demographic descriptors b. health problems both major and minor c. usual source of medical care d. level of satisfaction with medical care e. perceived health care needs of the community, i.e., ambulatory care facility, prevention programs		

Type	Relevance	Source of information
Subjective data:		
10. *Community's perception of itself* Informal gathering of data through interviews or discussions: a. individual's self-perception b. individual's view of community as a whole (Klein, 1982)		

Turn to the following pages to compare your answers.
a. relevance of data – p. 63
b. source of information – p. 63

SECTION 5.4

Two months have passed. You and your colleague have gathered data for nine of the ten categories listed in the previous section. *The board of directors has requested that a community survey/questionnaire not be conducted because of financial constraints.*

You and your colleague are preparing to present your findings, assessment, and recommendations to the agency director and the board of directors. You have summarized your findings as follows:

Objective Data:

Your observations of the community. Middletown is an upper-middle-class residential community of 15,000 located near the city of Boston. The size of Middletown grew rapidly over a ten-year period with extensive housing developments surrounding the original village. Despite this rapid growth, Middletown has retained its rural nature and remains a picturesque New England town with many large Colonial homes and traditional white steepled churches.

Middletown's population, which is primarily white Anglo-Saxon, consists of two groups, i.e., older, well-established families who are lifelong residents and younger families who have moved to Middletown to take advantage of its rural nature and the relatively short commuting distance to Boston. (Hadeka & Sutherland, 1977)

Geographical description of the community. Middletown covers an area of approximately 60 square miles; terrain is hilly. Access to Middletown is by winding two-lane highways; two major highways within ten miles of Middletown provide easy access to Boston. Middletown's primary natural resource is its close proximity to the metropolitan Boston area.

The majority of Middletown residents live in quiet neighborhoods of spacious, well-landscaped, single-dwelling homes.

The climate in the Middletown/Boston area is characterized by four distinct seasons. The average temperature is 58 °F; average summer temperature is 78 °F; average winter temperature is 33 °F. (Hadeka & Sutherland, 1977)

Descriptors of the population. (To help give additional significance to the population descriptors you have compared them with similar statistics for the city of Boston.)

The population of Middletown grew from 5,000 to 15,000 in ten years but has remained stable for the past five to six years. The median age of Middletown residents is 22; the median age in Boston is 28.9. The median income in Middletown is $24,000, substantially higher than the median income of $15,000 in Boston. Of the adult population, 41 percent have completed college compared with 15 percent in Boston. The majority of the adult population do not work in Middletown but travel to the metropolitan Boston area to work in professional and managerial roles, basically white-collar jobs.

The divorce rate in Middletown is slightly higher than in Boston, as is the remarriage rate.

The crime rate is substantially lower in Middletown than in Boston, but the rate of arrests in the adult population for DWI (driving while intoxicated) is slightly higher than that of Boston. (Hadeka & Sutherland, 1977)

Community services. With the growth of Middletown came the expansion of community services. New housing developments have access to the town water supply for consumption and fire protection. The town water supply comes from a nearby lake. With the growth in population, a water treatment plant was built that provides chlorination as well as fluoridation. It seems to be adequately meeting the needs of the town.

A sewage disposal plant was constructed in the 1970s and is meeting the needs of the town.

Shopping facilities have grown inconsistently. Although there are some businesses in the original village of Middletown, the majority, i.e., discount store, furniture store, supermarket, restaurants, and other small businesses, are located in two shopping centers in the newer sections of Middletown. The shopping centers are not easily accessible on foot; primary access is by car. Public transportation is limited to two daily buses that travel to and from Boston. (Hadeka & Sutherland, 1977)

Community resources. Middletown has three elementary schools, two of which were built since 1970 in the sections of town where new neighborhoods have been established. A large union high school to which students are bussed is located three miles from town. Each school has a part-time school nurse on contract from the home health agency who provides first aid, screening procedures, and formal as well as informal health education to individuals and groups. Each school has large, well-equipped playgrounds including tennis courts that are used by the children and townspeople year-round.

There are two large licensed day care centers, both functioning slightly below capacity. There is space available for additional children.

There is one subsidized housing unit for the elderly in Middletown that has not been filled to capacity in the five years it has been available. The home health agency does provide on-site services (two hours twice a week). Services include blood pressure screening, health counseling, and nutrition education.

There is one subsidized housing unit for low-income residents near one of the two shopping centers. It houses fifteen families. At present there is no waiting list of families requesting residency. (Hadeka & Sutherland, 1977)

Health resources. The health resources in Middletown are as follows:

Hospitals. There are no hospitals in Middletown. However, there are hospitals in three of the nearby towns (two small community hospitals, one large medical center); services provided are crisis oriented; distance to each hospital is 10-12 miles.

Emergency services. There is a volunteer ambulance service; the volunteers are certified EMT's and are individuals who work in Middletown; several are volunteer firemen. Emergency room services are located in two nearby towns each approximately 12 miles away. A review of a sample of emergency room admissions revealed that Middletown residents did not use emergency room services extensively but when used, the use was appropriate, i.e., fractures, musculoskeletal injuries.

Physicians. There are two physicians who practice medicine in Middletown. One is an internist and one a pediatrician.

Home health agency. Provides the services as described by the agency director on the first page of this Situation.

Mental health programs. There is one psychologist who practices in Middletown; his caseload primarily involves work with children and marriage counseling; there are several mental health programs in neighboring communities 10-12 miles away.

Self-help groups. Alcoholics Anonymous meets three evenings a week in Middletown; average attendance is 10-15 individuals.

Health clubs. There is one private health club in Middletown which has been in existence two years and has a large membership. The club offers tennis, racquet ball, swimming, and aerobic exercise classes. Health and nutritional counseling are not available; weekday clients average 125 per day; weekends 250 per day.

State health programs. Several serving maternal-child health clients in Middletown but no state services located directly in Middletown.

Pharmacy. There are two pharmacies, one located in Middletown village, another in one of the newer shopping centers.

Nursing homes. None located in Middletown, several within 10-15 miles.

With the majority of the adult population employed in professional and/or managerial positions outside Middletown (in the metropolitan Boston area), it might be assumed that these individuals and their families are receiving health care through one of the local physicians or a health maintenance organization by contractual arrangements with their employers. The type of health care sought is another unknown, indicating that *more data are needed.* (Hadeka & Sutherland, 1977)

Morbidity/mortality statistics. Morbidity statistics are difficult to find. One statistic that was available was the result of a community-wide hypertension screening and follow-up program done by the home health agency. The American Heart Association projects that at any screening program, 15 percent of those screened will be newly detected hypertensives; the screening in Middletown detected 30 percent, or twice that projected by the Heart Association.

Mortality statistics revealed that when compared with other towns in Massachusetts of the same size, Middletown residents were generally healthier. There were, however, two exceptions, which you have depicted in Figures 7 and 8. (Hadeka & Sutherland, 1977)

Community power structure. Middletown is governed by a board of selectmen composed of three lifelong residents of Middletown and four community members who have lived in Middletown for less than ten years. For many years, with the rapid growth of the town, there was a significant conflict in ideas among the new- and old-family members of the board of selectmen. The town manager, hired by the selectmen, has attempted to engage the selectmen and community members in long-range community planning.

In addition to the town officials, power seems to emanate from several large landholders, businessmen, and lawyers. (Hadeka & Sutherland, 1977)

Community survey/questionnaire. Information about the town of Middletown that could be obtained through a formal survey is not available because of financial constraints placed upon this assessment by the home health agency's board of directors.

Subjective Data:

Community's perception of itself. Middletown residents view their community as a relatively new middle-class American town with access to almost all services to meet their contemporary needs, e.g., cultural opportunities, medical technology, educational resources.

Based upon the data presented, in the work space provided:

    a. State your assessment of the community of Middletown.
    b. List the recommendations you will make to the home health agency's board of directors. Support your recommendations with rationale.

Student Work Space

Turn to the following pages to compare your answers.
a. assessment – p. 66
b. recommendations – p. 67

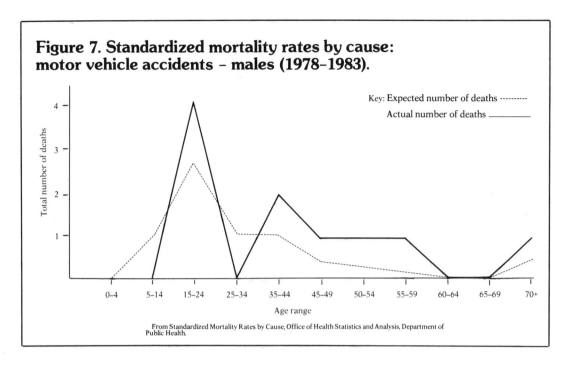

Figure 7. Standardized mortality rates by cause: motor vehicle accidents – males (1978–1983).

Key: Expected number of deaths ----------
Actual number of deaths _____

From Standardized Mortality Rates by Cause, Office of Health Statistics and Analysis, Department of Public Health.

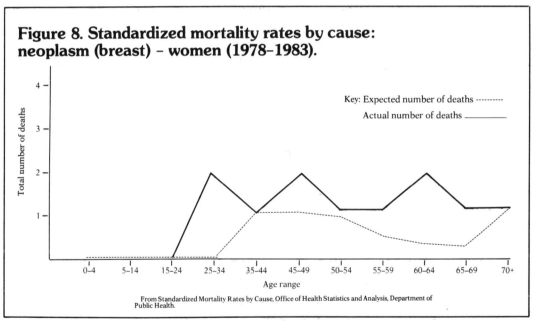

Figure 8. Standardized mortality rates by cause: neoplasm (breast) – women (1978–1983).

Key: Expected number of deaths ----------
Actual number of deaths _____

From Standardized Mortality Rates by Cause, Office of Health Statistics and Analysis, Department of Public Health.

ANSWERS TO SECTION 5.1

a. Should the board of directors support the proposal?

If you said that the board of directors should not support the agency director's proposal, you have made the right judgment. Although the director has presented reasons why an ambulatory care facility for the adult population might be appropriate, the rationale as presented in this situation is based on conjecture and intuition, not on objective data.

When developing a health care plan for an individual client, conjecture and intuition *may* come into play. However, the most appropriate plan of care is based on analysis of a complete data base consisting of both subjective and objective data.

This approach is even more important when planning for the health care needs of a total community, where the factors are much more complex. Planning based on an assessment of a comprehensive data base is the only basis for sound program development (Spradley, 1985; Higgs & Gustafson, 1985).

The director's proposal for an ambulatory care facility would have validity only if it could be supported with concrete objective data.

b. How do you think the board of directors should proceed?

You are absolutely right if you said the board of directors should *request additional data* before making a decision to support the establishment of an ambulatory care facility. Once data are gathered and analyzed, an accurate assessment can be made. Based upon the assessment, the agency director and the board of directors can make an informed decision.

In this situation the board of directors can proceed with one of two types of assessment:

    1. A comprehensive community assessment.
    2. An assessment of the health care needs of the adult population.
(Spradley, 1985)

The following questions may arise here: "Who would gather the data?" "Who would do the community assessment?" "Is such a role appropriate for the community health nurse?" Participation in a community assessment is indeed an appropriate role for the community health nurse. Unfortunately, it is a role about which the majority of community health nurses do not have extensive knowledge or actual experience. Planning for the health care needs of a community (or aggregate) generally occurs within the administrative ranks of an agency or institution by staff prepared for such roles through graduate education. As a result, the staff nurse involved in the day-to-day care of clients and families may be unaware of the community health planning done by others within the same agency (Williams, 1984).

While planning for the health care needs of a community may seem to many staff nurses like an insurmountable task, the conceptual framework used is the same problem-solving method used in the nursing process to plan for the health care needs of the individual client, i.e., gathering data to make an assessment, planning, implementation, and evaluation (Spradley, 1985; Higgs & Gustafson, 1985; Hall & Weaver, 1985).

ANSWERS TO SECTION 5.2 ————————————

a. Define community.

Define community: a simple request but not a simple task. The term *community* is consistently used by community health professionals in their practice, yet they define the term in widely different ways. Definitions range from broad and comprehensive to narrow and specific. Here are general definitions of community:

> "A collection of people who share some important feature of their lives" (Spradley, 1985, p. 5).

> "People in relationship to one another are the essential element of a community. In most communities, place is one of the strongest elements holding people together. However, in other communities, a common goal, a common perspective, or a common need provides the 'glue' of the relationship" (Hanchett, 1979, p. 10).

If your definition is similar to either of the above definitions, you are grasping the concept of community. If your definition is more specific than those given above, that's okay! Continue reading, as you may find your definition is similar to one of the following.

Archer and Fleshman (1985) have divided the types of communities into three categories for a clearer delineation of the various relationships that may comprise a community:

1. *Emotional communities* that develop around a sense or a feeling of community (ibid., p. 100).
2. *Structural communities* that involve time and space relationships between people (ibid., p. 102).
3. *Functional communities* that have a common belief by the people that community is whatever sense of the local common good citizens can be helped to achieve (ibid., p. 104).

These three categories encompass several different types of communities; the following chart briefly outlines the types of communities in each category, how they are defined, and some examples of each.

EMOTIONAL COMMUNITIES

Type	Definition (Archer & Fleshman, 1985)	Examples
Belonging community	A place where you are known and feel you belong	Hometown, high school, college, sorority
Special-interest community	A coalition whose members share a common interest or need	Mothers Against Drunk Drivers, Coalition for Peace

STRUCTURAL COMMUNITIES

Type	Definition (Archer & Fleshman, 1985)	Examples
Total community	An institution that provides for the needs of its members, thus eliminating outside contact	Prisons, mental institutions, religious cults
Face-to-face community	A community of members who are close to one another; know each other's problems; readily help one another	Families, neighborhoods, ethnic neighborhoods
Community of problem ecology	A geographical area whose residents are affected by an ecological problem	A town contaminated by mercury poisoning from an industry manufacturing thermometers; communities destroyed by forest fires

(continued)

STRUCTURAL COMMUNITIES (continued)

Type	Definition (Archer & Fleshman, 1985)	Examples
Geopolitical community	An area with clean geographical boundaries and political jurisdiction	Villages, towns, cities, counties, states
Organization	A group having some power and authority over the people it serves	Health departments, churches, private clubs
Community of solution	A community unit whose members work towards the resolution of a defined problem by identifying appropriate resources and personnel	School district; health district; health systems agencies

FUNCTIONAL COMMUNITIES

Type	Definition (Archer & Fleshman, 1985)	Examples
Community of identifiable need	A group whose members have a common problem and common needs	The pregnant adolescent population in a given city or county; industrial workers exposed to harmful chemicals
Critical mass community	Similar to community of solution; ad hoc in nature; resources and personnel are readily available to solve the problem	Community members find resources for high school athletes, i.e., the school with tennis courts shares them with a school that has a swimming pool; election committees; hospital expansion planning committee

b. Define community assessment.

If your definition of community assessment is similar to either of the following, good for you!

> "Community assessment is the initial step in the problem-solving process used to promote the health of a community" (Higgs & Gustafson, 1985, p. 17).

Community assessment is the process of gathering and analyz-
ing all data relevant to the health of the community. Based
upon the analysis of data, recommendations are made.

If you wonder why completion of a community assessment is essential, Higgs and
Gustafson (1985) identify the following five reasons for completing a community
assessment:

1. *Needs identification.* Community health needs and/or problems that
   may not be apparent may be identified once data are analyzed.
2. *Problem clarification.* A problem that has been identified may require additional data gathered before plans for resolving the problem can be formulated.
3. *Desire analysis.* Community members may express concern regarding an actual/potential community health problem; the community
   members request an assessment to substantiate their concerns.
4. *Resource identification.* Community health resources are identified
   and their services outlined; the information is then used by community agencies to avoid duplication of services within the community.
5. *Resource utilization.* Community health services are reviewed to determine whether or not their services are being used as intended.

ANSWERS TO SECTION 5.3

**a. Describe the relevance that the data in each of the ten major categories have in
the community assessment.**

b. State where you think the data in each of the categories can be found.

Type of data	Relevance	Source of information
Your observations of the community	Give the investigator an unbiased look at the community before data are gathered. Once data are gathered, the assessment may reveal a community quite different from the one seen during this cursory look.	Your objective observations when walking/driving around the community
Geographical description of the community	May be directly related to objective data gathered; e.g., winding roads may contribute to the number of automobile accidents, and hilly terrain and freezing temperatures in winter may contribute to the incidence of injuries resulting from falls.	Atlas; maps of town/city, county, state; town/city report; town/city government; public library, chamber of commerce, personal observations

(continued)

Type of data	Relevance	Source of information
Descriptors of the population	Give the investigator a general description of the total population for which recommendations will be made. Recommendations should take the descriptors into consideration; e.g., recommendations for an ethnic population should take ethnic tradition into account. The remaining descriptors of the population, i.e., unemployment, crime, are stress indicators; give the investigator data on how much and what type of stress the community has compared with similar communities.	U.S. census data, state health department, town/city government, chamber of commerce, U.S. Department of Labor Statistics
Community services	Identify what the community has/needs/can afford, explore lack of services which in some situations may be directly related to health problems; e.g., a low-income neighborhood may not have the same sewage disposal facilities as the rest of the community, and this could be directly related to recurrent epidemics in the neighborhood.	Chamber of commerce, city/town government, city/town directory, telephone book, community members
Community resources	Identify what the community has and/or needs, identify over/under utilization of services. Data used when making recommendations, e.g., avoiding duplication of services or encouraging reallocation of resources.	Chamber of commerce, city/town government, city/town directory, telephone book, community agencies, community members
Health resources	Identify what the community has and/or	Chamber of commerce,

Type of data	Relevance	Source of information
Health resources	needs, explore for over/under use of specific health resources. Data used when making recommendations, e.g., avoiding duplication of services, encouraging reallocation of resources, or recommending different approaches to facilitate use of resources.	city/town government, city/town directory, telephone book, community agencies, health planning boards, community members
Morbidity/mortality statistics	Identify what the major health problems are in the community. Objective data documenting the causes of death in a community are indisputable. Such statistics may not be noted by the community as a whole or by community agencies; e.g., the number of deaths caused by stroke in a particular community may be significantly higher than that in similar communities.	State health department, town/city clerk's office
Community power structure	Identifies key individuals in the community. Having these individuals identified may be essential when attempting to implement recommendations because influential community members have been known to sabotage an appropriate health care program for various reasons—failure to understand the program, lack of involvement in the planning, etc. Gaining the support of key community individuals could instead enlist their support of the recommendations made.	Community library, town/city government, community agencies, community members

(continued)

Type of data	*Relevance*	*Source of information*
Community survey/ question- naire	Gives the investigator some objective data from the community members describing themselves, their health problems, and their needs. When sum- marized, these data are compared with other objective data col- lected. Data collection by means of a question- naire is more reliable than an informal, man- on-the-street survey.	Community mem- bers who have selected to participate in the survey by ran- dom sampling
Community's perception of itself	Gives the investigator some understanding of the community as a whole; i.e.: Is this a friendly town? Are in- dividuals interested in the welfare of their community? Note that these data are subjec- tive in nature and can- not be generalized to the community as a whole; the time of day and location selected for interviewing indi- viduals may affect the responses obtained.	Community agencies, community members

ANSWERS TO SECTION 5.4

a. State your assessment of the community of Middletown.

1. Most of the adult population of Middletown have access to health care resources in nearby communities for emergency situations. These services are used appropriately. The adult population of Mid- dletown have access to health care resources through health main- tenance organizations associated with their place of employment.
2. Middletown is an affluent, well-educated community whose resi- dents are generally healthier than residents in communities of sim- ilar size with three exceptions:
   a. The incidence of individuals with newly detected hypertension is twice the rate projected by the American Heart Association.
   b. The number of deaths in the male population from motor vehicle accidents was above that projected by the state, as shown in Fig- ure 7.
   c. The number of deaths in the female population from breast cancer was above that projected by the state, as shown in Figure 8.

3. Community services and resources have expanded with the population of Middletown and are adequately meeting the needs of the residents.
4. A community of 15,000 residents cannot be expected to provide residents with an extensive range of health resources; the health resources available in the town of Middletown and nearby communities seem to provide for the needs of the population with one exception: the only community health programs within Middletown having a focus on prevention are the hypertension screening program and prenatal care classes. (Hadeka & Sutherland, 1977)

If your assessment of the community of Middletown is similar to the above assessment, you can be proud of yourself. As you can see from sifting through the data collected for the community assessment, the areas of concern for the health of this community are areas that could easily go unrecognized as health problems by the majority of community members.

If your assessment of the community of Middletown is not similar to the above assessment, take time to go back and reevaluate the data gathered, which do provide an accurate portrayal of the health of this community.

b. List the recommendations you will make to the home health agency's board of directors. Support your recommendations with rationale.

Based upon the summary of the data collected, the following recommendations are appropriate. If your recommendations and rationale are similar, you have a good understanding of what would be appropriate for the community of Middletown.

Recommendations (Hadeka & Sutherland, 1977)	*Rationale*
1. A community health center to serve the adult population of Middletown is not recommended.	1. As the data show, the adult population have access to health care resources for both acute and nonacute problems with an internist and pediatrician practicing in town. Community residents also have access to emergency facilities in nearby communities and health maintenance organizations. The establishment of such a health care facility would only duplicate existing resources.
2. A comprehensive program focusing on prevention should be developed and implemented by an existing community agency, specifically the Middletown Home Health Care Agency. Preven-	2. The major statistics that stand out in this community assessment are the high incidence of hypertension, the deaths from breast cancer, and the deaths from motor vehicle accidents. All of these are preventable. The hypertension and motor vehicle deaths can easily be related to life-style; 75 percent of the deaths of North Americans can be attributed to life-style (LaLonde, 1974, p. 33).

(continued)

Recommendations
(Hadeka & Sutherland,
1977)

tion programs
should address the
following:
a. Effects of
   American life-
   style on health
b. Stress reduc-
   tion
c. Smoking
   cessation
d. Effects of
   American diet
   on health
e. Self breast
   examination
f. Self testicular
   examination
g. Accident
   prevention,
   i.e., motor
   vehicle, house-
   hold, bicycle,
   athletic
h. Alcohol and
   drug use

Rationale

Hypertension, which increases the likelihood of heart disease and stroke, plays a major role in premature disability of adult workers (Starck, 1984). Programs designed for hypertensive clients have been effective in assisting individuals with stress reduction, smoking cessation, and dietary changes (Lowther & Carter, 1981). With the incidence of hypertension in the community, community members need to be educated regarding its causes and risks.

Stress is a contributing factor to hypertension and is often a product of the American life-style. While everyone experiences stressful situations, ways of dealing with stress vary greatly. Those who suffer negative consequences from stress can benefit from programs that will help them identify constructive and healthy ways to deal with the stress and/or stressor, i.e., meditation, visual imagery, biofeedback, muscle relaxation exercises, improvement in communication patterns.

Cancer of the breast is the most common malignancy in American women, affecting 1 in 13 women (Public Health Service, 1979). Heredity is considered a factor. The impact of environmental and behavioral factors is not clear (Public Health Service, 1979). Early detection is essential. All women need to be convinced of the value of self breast examination and shown the correct way to do it.

Motor vehicle accidents were the leading cause of death in the United States in 1977 in the 15-24 year age group, accounting for 37 percent of all deaths. In the adult population motor vehicle accidents are also a leading cause of death (Public Health Service, 1979). *Fifty percent* of all drivers involved in fatal accidents are found to have excessive blood alcohol levels (Public Health Service,

1979). A comprehensive community program for reducing motor vehicle accidents could be offered by the home health agency in conjunction with health educators and driver education instructors from the public school system.

3. The existing hypertension screening program should be maintained.

3. See rationale for hypertension above. In addition, clients involved in the hypertension screening program can be referred to the programs on stress reduction, smoking cessation, and nutrition as indicated by their needs.

4. Members of the board of directors of the Middletown Home Health Care Agency should share the findings of this assessment with influential community members to gain their support in implementing prevention programs.

4. Gaining the support of influential community members will increase the likelihood that the prevention programs will be accepted by the community members.

5. Members of the board of directors of the Middletown Home Health Care Agency should share these findings with school board officials and encourage the integration of the prevention programs listed in #2 into the Middletown school system.

5. Although the school-age population is relatively healthy, the issue of lifestyle remains. Introducing children and adolescents to the concepts of prevention and health promotion may lead to an even healthier adult population in the future.

Resolution

The summary of the community assessment data and the recommendations were presented to the Middletown Home Health Care Agency board of directors and the agency director. The response from the group was unexpected. Despite the statistics presented, the board of directors and the agency director continued to express their belief that there was a need for a health care center in Middletown to meet the needs of the adult population. They acknowledged that the idea of a prevention-focused program was interesting but questioned whether Middletown residents would pay for and participate in such a program.

As a result, the board of directors asked the two community health nurses who had completed the assessment to proceed with a community-wide survey. The nurses developed a questionnaire to be sent to adult heads of household asking for the following information:

- a. Demographic descriptors.
- b. Health problems they faced during the past year, i.e., both minor ailments and major health problems.
- c. Source of medical care.
- d. Level of satisfaction with medical care.
- e. Perceived health care needs of the community, i.e., ambulatory care facility, prevention programs.

In addition, community members were asked if, given a choice of preventive programs (many were listed), they would use the programs and would be willing to pay for the programs.

The town directory was used and families were assigned numbers. A table of random numbers was then used to select the random sample to whom the questionnaires were sent.

The results of the survey indicated that the demographic characteristics of the residents were as described in the community assessment. In addition, the survey revealed that Middletown residents were extremely healthy. They stated that they did have easy access to medical care primarily through health maintenance organizations in the metropolitan Boston area and that they did not think a health care center for the adult population was needed in Middletown.

The response to the preventive programs was overwhelmingly positive, and residents said they would be willing to pay for them.

The community health nurses' recommendations from the community assessment were then reexamined, and a two-year timetable was outlined for implementation of all of the recommendations.

References

Archer, S. E., & Fleshman, R. P. (1985). *Community health nursing.* (3d ed.) Belmont, CA: Wadsworth.

Burgess, A. W. (1976). Lecture. Chestnut Hill, MA: Boston College.

Goeppinger, J. (1984). Community as client: Using the nursing process to promote health. In M. Stanhope & J. Lancaster (Eds.). *Community health nursing.* St. Louis: Mosby (pp. 379–404).

Hadeka, M. A., & Sutherland, J. (1977). Community assessment: An unpublished paper. Chestnut Hill, MA: Boston College.

Hall, J. E., & Weaver, B. R. (1985). *A systems approach to community health.* (2d ed.) Philadelphia: Lippincott.

Hanchett, E. S. (1979). *Community health assessment: A conceptual tool kit.* New York: Wiley.

Higgs, Z. R., & Gustafson, D. D. (1985). *Community as a client: Assessment and diagnosis.* Philadelphia: Davis.

Klein, D. C. (1982). Assessing community characteristics. In B. W. Spradley (Ed.). *Readings in community health nursing.* (2d ed.) Boston: Little, Brown (pp. 145–153).

LaLonde, M. (1974). *New perspectives on the health of Canadians.* Ottawa, Canada: Government Printing House.

Lowther, N. B., & Carter, V. D. (1981). How to increase compliance in hypertensives. *American Journal of Nursing* 81 (5):963.

Public Health Service (1979). *Healthy people: The surgeon general's report on health promotion and disease prevention* (DHEW Publication No. 79-55071). Washington, DC: U.S. Government Printing Office.

Rodgers, S. S. (1984). Community as client—a multivariate model for analysis of community and aggregate health risk. *Public Health Nursing* 1(4):210–222.

Spradley, B. W. (1985). *Community health nursing: Concepts and practice.* (2d ed.) Boston: Little, Brown.

Starck, P. (1984). Major community health problems of young and middle adults. In M. Stanhope & J. Lancaster (Eds.). *Community health nursing.* St. Louis: Mosby (pp. 621–647).

Williams, C. A. (1984). Population-focused practice. In M. Stanhope & J. Lancaster (Eds.). *Community health nursing.* St. Louis: Mosby (pp. 805–815).

PART II

School Health

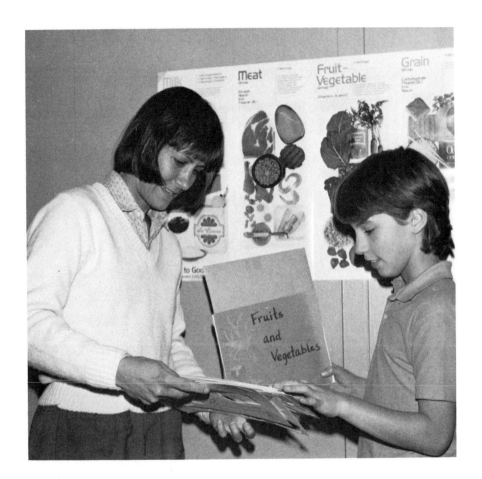

~~~ SITUATION 6 ~~~
Assessment of the School-Age Child
~~~ (Group Discussion) ~~~

SECTION 6.1 _____

You are the nurse at Springfield Elementary School. It is a rainy spring morning. John, a five-year-old, arrives in your office with a note in his hand written by the kindergarten teacher:

> Mrs. Smith,
>   Please check John. I don't think he feels well, yet he denies feeling sick. His attention span has been poor for the last two days, and he acts tired.
>   Thank you,
>   Mrs. Jones

John does look tired; he is pale and has dark circles under his eyes. He sits quietly on the bed in your office while you pull his health record from your file. His record states that John has a history of asthma and is allergic to a variety of flowering plants.

In the work space provided:

   a. List the parameters you will address in your assessment of John.
   b. State your rationale for the parameters you have selected.

Student Work Space _____

SECTION 6.2

Clinical Findings

To be read by faculty member.

In the work space provided:

    a. State your assessment.
    b. What do you think would be appropriate outcome(s) for John?
    c. Briefly outline a plan to help John reach the outcome(s) you have
       identified.

Student Work Space

SECTION 6.3

New Information

To be read by faculty member.

In the work space provided:

    a. Identify whom you would call and why.
    b. Identify what information you will relay to that person.
    c. Identify what recommendation you will make to that person.

Student Work Space

SECTION 6.4

Clinical Findings

Additional information to be read by faculty member.

In the work space provided:

a. List what parameters you would address in your assessment of John.

b. State your rationale for the parameters you have selected.

Student Work Space

SECTION 6.5

Clinical Findings

To be given by faculty member.

In the work space provided:

  a. State your assessment.
  b. Briefly outline a plan of care for John.
  c. Is follow-up appropriate? State your rationale.

Student Work Space

Suggested Reading

American Academy of Pediatrics (1981). *School health: A guide for professionals.* Evanston, IL: Author.

Clemen, S. A., Eigsti, D. G., & McGuire, S. L. (1981). *Comprehensive family and community health nursing.* New York: McGraw-Hill.

Coletta, S. S. (1978). Values clarification in nursing: Why? *American Journal of Nursing* 78(12):2057.

Fry, S. T. (1985). Values clarification in nursing: Application to practice. In B. W. Spradley (Ed.). *Community health nursing.* (2d ed.) Boston: Little, Brown (pp. 106–128).

Hahn, A. B., Barkin, R. L., & Oestreich, S. J. K. (1982). *Pharmacology in nursing.* (15th ed.) St. Louis: Mosby.

Malasanos, L., Barkauskas, V., Moss, M., & Stoltenberg-Allen, K. (1981). *Health assessment.* (2d ed.) St. Louis: Mosby.

Pohl, M. L. (1968). *Teaching function of the nursing practitioner.* Dubuque, IA: Brown.

Scipien, G. N., Barnard, M. U., Chard, M. A., Howe, J., & Phillips, P. J. (1979). *Comprehensive pediatric nursing.* (2d ed.) New York: McGraw-Hill.

Sheridan, E., Patterson, H. R., & Gustafson, E. A. (1982). *Falconer's The drug, the nurse, the patient.* (7th ed.) Philadelphia: Saunders.

Stuart, G. W., & Sundeen, S. J. (1983). *Principles and practice of psychiatric nursing.* (2d ed.) St. Louis: Mosby.

Uttecht, J. (1983). Teaching children responsibility for health. *Vermont Registered Nurse,* January 1983, 5–6.

Uustal, D. (1978). Values clarification in nursing: Application to practice. *American Journal of Nursing* 78(12):2058–2063.

Whaley, L. F., & Wong, D. L. (1983). *Nursing care of infants and children.* (2d ed.) St. Louis: Mosby.

Wold, S. J. (1981). *School nursing: A framework for practice.* St. Louis: Mosby.

SITUATION 7
The Playground Accident
(Self-Paced)

SECTION 7.1

You are the nurse at Arthur J. Rhodes School (grades K-8). It is early Tuesday morning and children are arriving at school. A seventh-grade girl comes running into your office and tells you there has been an accident at the edge of the playground. She says a boy in her class rode his bicycle down a steep embankment and hit a large log. She thinks his leg is broken. You plan to go to the accident site immediately.

In the work space provided:

    a. List what equipment (if any) you will take with you.

Student Work Space

Turn to the following page and compare your answer.
a. equipment – p. 85

SECTION 7.2

When you arrive at the site of the accident you find the following:

Mark, a 12-year-old boy, has ridden his bicycle down a steep embankment. When his bicycle hit a large log at the bottom, Mark was thrown over the handlebars and landed about ten feet away. He is sitting upright supporting himself with his arms. He is crying loudly that his right leg is broken. There are two teachers and a large crowd of children clustered around Mark.

In the work space provided:

    a. List the subjective data you will address in assessing Mark, and state your rationale for selecting them.
    b. List the objective data you will address in assessing Mark, and state your rationale for selecting them.
    c. Identify what comfort measures (if any) you will provide for Mark.
    d. Identify what you will do regarding the teachers and the crowd of children around Mark.

Student Work Space

Turn to the following pages and compare your answers.
    a. subjective data and rationale – p. 86
    b. objective data and rationale – p. 87
    c. comfort measures – p. 88
    d. crowd of children – p. 88

SECTION 7.3

Clinical Findings

When you assess Mark, you find the following: Mark says the only place he has pain is in the bottom part of his right leg. Mark says he landed on his right leg. He says he knows it's broken because he "heard and felt it snap." He says he did not land on his back and did not hit his head. He is clenching his fists and says he can see blood on his sock.

Mark's color is good. His skin is warm and dry. He is obviously alert and oriented. He states he did not hit his head. His pupils are equal and reactive to light. You carefully cut his jeans away from his leg. As you look at his leg there is an area of swelling approximately 3 in. in diameter midway between his knee and ankle. The surrounding tissue is rapidly becoming ecchymotic. Approximately 8 in. above his ankle is an open wound with a ragged configuration about 1½ in. in length from which a small piece of bone is protruding. The wound is bleeding. There appear to be approximately 30 cc of blood on his sock.

Based upon the above findings, in the work space provided:

   a. State your assessment.
   b. List the immediate steps to be taken to ensure rapid transport of Mark to an emergency room.
   c. Briefly describe the care you will provide for Mark.
   d. What level of prevention are you practicing—primary, secondary, or tertiary?

Student Work Space

Turn to the following pages and compare your answers.
   a. assessment – p. 89
   b. immediate steps – p. 89
   c. care – p. 90
   d. level of prevention – p. 91

SECTION 7.4

As you are giving the principal (or teacher) the information to be relayed to the rescue squad and Mark's parents, Mark interrupts you and tells you that his parents are away on vacation. He and his sister have been staying with an aunt and uncle. Both work nearby.

In the work space provided:

> a. State who should be called.
> b. List what information should be relayed to the individual(s) notified.
> c. State the recommendations you will make to the individual(s).

Student Work Space

Turn to the following pages and compare your answers.
  a. who should be called – p. 91
  b. information to be relayed – p. 91
  c. recommendations – p. 92

SECTION 7.5

Mark's uncle arrives at the school within a few minutes. He says his wife is trying to contact Mark's parents. Within another few minutes, the ambulance arrives. You give the rescue squad a quick, concise description of what has happened and what you have done. Mark is then taken to the hospital; his uncle accompanies him in the ambulance.

You return to your office. A teacher comes in and tells you he thinks you handled Mark's care efficiently and effectively. He comments that you must be relieved that it is over.

In the work space provided answer the following:

> a. What is an assertive response to the teacher's comment?
> b. Is this situation one that warrants an accident report? If no, why? If yes, list the type of information you feel is appropriate to include.
> c. Is follow-up appropriate in this situation? If no, why? If yes, state your rationale.

Student Work Space

Turn to the following pages and compare your answers.
a. assertive response – p. 92
b. accident report – p. 92
c. follow-up – p. 93

ANSWERS TO SECTION 7.1

a. Equipment

The following equipment could be taken to the accident site by the school nurse:

Splint – for immobilization of the affected limb if indeed a fracture exists.

Blanket – to provide coverage for maintaining body temperature in the event the child does have a fracture and is experiencing early signs of shock.

Pillow – to provide comfort for the child if he does have to be immobilized.

First-aid kit – to care for any cuts, bruises, or lacerations.

Scissors – to remove clothing from the affected limb while keeping the limb immobilized.

Paper/pen – for documentation.

If you indicated you would not take equipment with you, your reasons might be the following:

- wastes valuable time
- cumbersome to carry
- don't really know what you'll need until the situation has been assessed

The above list is lengthy, and if items are not consolidated they could be cumbersome to carry. Consolidation could be part of preplanning for accident management by the school nurse. For example: *splint* – store with a lightweight *blanket* and small *pillow* attached; *first-aid kit* – keep well stocked, with *scissors* inside. With these items easily accessible the nurse has used time efficiently and can approach the accident site well prepared.

What comprises a well-stocked first-aid kit?

First-aid kits can be assembled by the individual nurse or purchased in a variety of sizes (depending on the situation and projected needs, i.e., for home use, for use within a school or a large company). A purchased kit contains a complete assortment of standard first-aid materials, clearly labeled and easy to locate.

The following is a list of contents in the 16-unit first-aid kit (American Red Cross, 1979, p. 223). First-aid kits also are sold in 24- or 32-unit kits.

> 2 units – 1-in. adhesive compress
> 2 units – 2-in. bandage compress
> 1 unit – 3-in. bandage compress
> 1 unit – 4-in. bandage compress
> 1 unit – 3-by-3-in. plain gauze
> 1 unit – gauze roller bandage
> 2 units – plain absorbent gauze, 1/2 sq yd
> 2 units – plain absorbent gauze, 24 by 72 in.
> 3 units – triangular bandage, 40 in.
> 1 unit – tourniquet, scissors, tweezers

If you are assembling your own first-aid kit, be certain that:

> 1. It is large enough to hold your materials.
> 2. You arrange items for easy access.
> 3. You wrap items to protect those not used from becoming dirty.
> (American Red Cross, 1979, p. 224)

ANSWERS TO SECTION 7.2 ─────────

A comprehensive data base is needed for you to make an accurate assessment of the injured child. Subjective data and objective data need to be obtained.

a. Subjective data and rationale

Subjective data	*Rationale* (American Red Cross, 1979; Long, 1983)
1. Where—and how much —does it hurt?	1. Pain will be immediate and severe at fracture site.
2. Can he move the affected limb?	2. Usually with a fracture the individual loses function of the affected limb.
3. Did he feel or hear the bone snap?	3. A common occurrence with fractures.
4. Does he feel a grating or rubbing sensation in the area of pain?	4. Rubbing or grating (crepitus) can occur if the bone fragments come in contact with one another. *No attempt should ever be made to elicit this symptom, as more damage will result.*
5. Does he feel movement	5. Displacement of the bones and/or

| where movement does not usually occur? | fragments can cause abnormal motion even when limb is not being moved. |

In the list of subjective data identified above, location/intensity of pain and loss of function are the most obvious complaints that the child will report. The remaining three are less obvious, and the nurse may need to elicit this information.

An additional piece of subjective data which you may have identified is how the accident happened. If you did identify this as information you would obtain, you are correct. It is valuable information; i.e., it becomes part of your nursing history, and knowing Mark's perception of what happened could enhance your assessment: e.g., "I was racing with . . . and lost control of my bike. . . . I flew over the handlebars and landed on my leg." If Mark gave information such as "I hit my head," then you would automatically assess his head/neck in depth. You are gathering subjective and objective data in addition to allowing Mark to express his feelings about the accident.

Based on the data you have, Mark's primary injury is his fractured leg. Your highest priorities are assessment, care, and stabilization of the child and his injury.

b. Objective data and rationale

To obtain the needed objective data in this situation, the nurse may need to cut the clothing away from the affected leg, *using extreme caution not to move the leg.*

Objective data	*Rationale* (American Red Cross, 1979; Long, 1983)
1. Vital signs, i.e., pulse, color, temperature, level of consciousness, respirations, pupillary response	1. If the injury is severe, the nurse should watch for signs of early shock at least every 15 minutes.
2. Difference in shape and length of corresponding bones in the other leg	2. The configuration of the affected leg may differ from that of the other leg if there has been displacement of the bone or bone fragments.
3. Obvious deformities	3. There will be gross deformity of the limb if there has been marked displacement of bone fragments.
4&5. Edema; hemorrhaging	4&5. Because bones are firmer than the surrounding structures, a fracture can injure the tissues, nerves, muscles, etc., causing edema and hemorrhaging into surrounding tissues (or external hemorrhaging).
6. Pain or tenderness to touch	6. Usually immediate and severe; aggravated by attempted movement.
7. Presence/absence of an open wound	7. An open wound will be present with a compound fracture (the bone may slip back under the skin).

It is possible for a fracture to occur with no displacement of fragments, minimal swelling, and pain only if direct pressure is applied. The fracture may be obvious only on x-ray.

The question may arise here regarding the gathering of subjective and objective data separately. Is it necessary? Can they be gathered simultaneously? As the nurse becomes more proficient at data gathering, subjective and objective data can be gathered simultaneously, thus increasing the efficiency of the nurse.

In emergency situations data have to be gathered quickly and thoroughly. A danger in the practice of gathering subjective and objective data simultaneously is that the nurse has a tendency to concentrate on his or her own observations (objective data) and not to hear everything the client says (subjective data).

In emergency situations one can easily forget to record data, e.g., pulse rate when taken initially. Recording data prevents their loss and enables comparison with later readings. If you cannot record the data yourself, assign someone to do it for you, such as one of the teachers nearby.

c. Comfort measures

Comfort measures for the injured person in any emergency situation can be beneficial in decreasing the apprehension/fear the individual may be experiencing. In this situation particularly, because the injured person is a child who is away from his major support systems (i.e., parents/family), it is crucial for him to feel secure and trust those caring for him. The following comfort measures would be appropriate in this situation (American Red Cross, 1979):

> *Touch Mark*; establish physical contact with him; have someone (a teacher/older student/sibling) maintain hand-to-hand contact with him.
> *Talk to Mark*; call him by name; assure him that you will remain with him; let him know he will be taken care of quickly; let him know it's all right for him to cry.
> Have him lie down (a small pillow can be placed under his head); this will help to decrease chances of early shock.
> Cover him with a blanket to maintain body temperature and help decrease chances of early shock.
> Do not move him.

If you indicated in your answer that you would not have instituted any comfort measures, your reasoning might have been that immediate care was of greater priority. Immediate care *is* the highest priority, but it can include comfort measures. In crisis situations, people need to feel that those caring for them are competent, and they need to hear sincere encouragement (American Red Cross, 1979, p. 17).

d. Crowd dispersal

Dispersing the crowd is the responsibility of the individual in charge of the emergency situation (American Red Cross, 1979); in this case, it is the school nurse. It can be done simultaneously while caring for the child by enlisting the assistance of the teachers at the accident site. Have one teacher stay with you to assist you in caring for Mark while the other takes charge of moving the crowd of children away. This is also an appropriate time to designate someone (an older student) to alert a school administrator, i.e., principal, assistant principal, to come to the accident site.

If you indicated in your answer that you would not be concerned with crowd dispersal, your reasoning might have been that care of the child was a higher priority. Although that is correct, providing efficient, effective care in the midst of a crowd is difficult even for the most experienced professional. The presence of a crowd can increase the stress level of the injured child as well as the individuals providing the care.

ANSWERS TO SECTION 7.3

a. Assessment

The open wound and protruding bone fragment indicate that this is a compound fracture, at risk for infection, shock, and further tissue damage.

b. Plan

To ensure rapid transport of Mark to an emergency room the following steps are suggested.

Immediate steps	*Rationale* (American Red Cross, 1979; Long, 1983)
1. Call for ambulance/rescue squad. Delegate a teacher/administrator to place a call for the rescue squad. Have them *address these questions*: Where is the emergency? Phone number? What happened? How many persons need help? What is being done?	1. A compound fracture is a priority for emergency transportation. Open fractures are considered more serious than closed ones because contamination of the fracture area puts the client at high risk for infection. A closed fracture and/or a suspected fracture should also be treated promptly, but there is less risk in delay.
2. Call child's family. Delegate a teacher/administrator to make the call for you. Have the individual identify which child is injured, what happened, and the extent of the injuries and give reassurance that the child is receiving appropriate care. Direct the parent to proceed to the hospital emergency room to meet the child when he arrives (particularly if the parent lives at a distance). If the parent lives/works close to the school, you may want him or her to come directly to the school.	2. You want to inform the parent, giving complete and accurate information. You want the parent to be with the child during this time of crisis to provide love, comfort, moral support, and consent for treatment. In each of the above instances the individual who makes the phone calls should remain calm and clear in conveying the information to avoid confusion and misinterpretation of information.

c. Care of Mark

Immediate steps	*Rationale* (American Red Cross, 1979; Long, 1983)
1. Cover open wound with a dry, sterile dressing from first-aid kit or a clean cloth. *Do not* clean wound. *Do not* probe wound. *Do not* apply pressure.	1. To keep as clean as possible. Because the bone has penetrated the skin, a portal of entry has been established and contamination of sterile tissue, i.e., bone, muscle, has occurred. The primary concern is to prevent further contamination. If a sterile dressing is not available, a clean dressing or clean cloth may be used to cover the open wound.
2. Control bleeding. Cover with dressing. In case of severe bleeding apply pressure at pressure point. *Do not* apply pressure at the site of the fracture.	2. To prevent shock from hemorrhage. Apply pressure at the pressure point above the fracture, i.e., popliteal space. If pressure is applied at the site of the fracture, extensive damage will be done to the bones and the surrounding tissue.
3. Since the rescue squad has been called, immobilize leg with blanket and pillow. If no rescue squad is available, immobilize leg with a splint. When splinting a fracture *splint the extremity as you find it. Exception:* severely angulated fractures of the *shafts* of bones of the extremities (Long, 1983, p. 1903). Do not attempt to reduce the fracture. Have teacher assist you with splinting. The teacher can hold splint; you can support joints above and below fracture. The splint should support these same joints.	3. To keep the ends of the fractured bone and adjacent joints from moving. Reduction should be done only by the medical staff once the child reaches the hospital. Splinting the leg will protect the leg from further damage.

The question may arise here, "*What would happen if the school nurse were not available to provide the above care?*" This is an excellent question, as there are times when the school nurse will not be available. The nurse can assist school officials by establishing a practice of informing them of his or her schedule and where he or she can be reached by telephone (American Academy of Pediatrics, 1981).

It is unrealistic to assume that the nurse will always be readily accessible, so the nurse should assume responsibility for establishing a plan for accident management in his or her absence. Obtaining administrative support for development of such a program will increase its effectiveness. Teachers and staff can be taught how to manage accidents effectively through in-service education programs offered by the nurse. Content of such programs can range in scope from the less serious accidents to the more complex.

d. Level of prevention

The level of prevention practiced in this situation would be *secondary prevention.* Secondary prevention begins once a problem has been identified.

Shamansky and Clausen (1980, p. 106) describe secondary prevention as "early diagnosis and prompt intervention to halt the pathological process, thereby shortening its duration and severity and enabling the individual to regain normal function at the earliest possible point. Early diagnosis is illustrated by the use of a comprehensive nursing assessment, which may reveal the need for further medical evaluation."

In the situation with Mark a problem has been identified; there is a compound fracture of his leg. Early diagnosis and prompt intervention are key concepts here. Early diagnosis (assessment) by the nurse was based upon a comprehensive data base derived from subjective and objective data. Prompt intervention (first aid) by the nurse involved providing immediate care for Mark at the accident site and arranging for him to be transported to an acute care facility for medical care.

If you selected tertiary prevention as the level of prevention being practiced, read the following definition of tertiary prevention by Shamansky and Clausen (1980, p. 106): "Tertiary prevention comes into play when a defect or disability is fixed, stabilized, or irreversible. Rehabilitation, the goal of tertiary prevention, is more than halting the disease process itself; it is restoring the individual to an optimum level of functioning within the constraints of the disability."

When you compare Mark's situation to the above definition there is no indication at this time that his compound fracture will result in a "fixed, stabilized, or irreversible" state.

ANSWERS TO SECTION 7.4 ——————————

a. Who should be called

Mark's aunt and uncle should be notified, as they are the individuals to whom the parents have given responsibility in their absence. Mark's parents should also be notified; however, school officials can relinquish that responsibility to the aunt and uncle. In addition, Mark's sister should be notified (if she is not already aware of the accident).

b. Information to be relayed

The information relayed to the aunt and uncle should be consistent with that previously identified, i.e., which child is injured, what happened, the extent of the injuries, reassurance that the child is receiving appropriate care, and how the child is being transported to the hospital.

This information should be given in a calm, clear fashion to avoid confusion and/or misinterpretation of the information by the aunt/uncle. Assurance that the child is receiving appropriate care will help decrease stress for the aunt/uncle.

c. Recommendations

Recommend that the aunt/uncle proceed to the hospital emergency room to meet the child on his arrival there (particularly if the adult resides/works at a distance). If the relative is within easy access of the school, recommend coming to the school to accompany the child to the hospital in the rescue vehicle.

Recommend that the aunt/uncle contact Mark's parents immediately. Because Mark's injuries are extensive he will require surgery, for which parental consent will be required. More important, at a time of crisis the child needs and wants his major support systems with him to provide the love, comfort, and security he needs.

ANSWERS TO SECTION 7.5

a. Assertive response

The response of the nurse to the teacher will vary depending upon the nurse's interpretation of the teacher's last statement: "You must be relieved that it's over." How did you interpret the statement—positively or negatively?

The nurse who interprets the teacher's comment as a positive expression of concern may feel free to discuss his or her feelings.

The nurse who interprets the teacher's statement as a putdown could respond in one of several ways:

1. By saying little or nothing because the teacher's comment seems to be a criticism of the way the situation was handled. This response would be *nonassertive* (Pointer & Lancaster, 1984).
2. By becoming angry or sarcastic and lashing out at the teacher. This response would be *aggressive* (Pointer & Lancaster, 1984).
3. By stating his or her feelings about the situation in a calm, thoughtful manner. This response would be *assertive* (Pointer & Lancaster, 1984). A variety of assertive statements would be appropriate in this situation:
   a. "I feel this morning's situation went smoothly with good cooperation from staff."
   b. "I feel good that Mark is safely on his way to the hospital."
   c. "I agree that things went well."
   d. "Thank you."

If you indicated above that you interpreted the teacher's statement as negative, what type of response do you think you would have made: nonassertive, aggressive, or assertive?

b. Accident report

An accident report is essential (Wold, 1979). Each school should have policies outlining when accident reports need to be completed and the specific type of information to be included in the report (Wold, 1979).

In any school accident report the following areas/questions should be addressed:

1. Name, age, and address of the child
2. Date, time, and location of accident
3. Description of the accident
4. Names of individuals who witnessed/described the accident
5. Description of the injury sustained

  6. Description of the care given to the child
  7. Disposition of the child, i.e., to home or hospital and with whom
  8. Name of the individual who delivered the care/prepared the accident report
  9. Name of parent(s)/guardian(s) contacted; date and time of contact

The information recorded should be concise but complete (American Academy of Pediatrics, 1981). It should be factual (objective) in nature. It should not contain inferences. The accident report will be kept on file at the school. Local school policy will determine whether it becomes a part of the child's school record.

The question of who pays the child's medical expenses may arise at this time. In most situations, the medical expenses will be paid through insurance coverage carried by the child's parents. Some schools offer optional insurance plans to parents which provide coverage if the child is injured during school hours and on school property.

In a situation such as this one with Mark, the possibility of a parent's filing suit against the school always exists. As a result, each school carries liability insurance. In addition, each principal, teacher, and school nurse may carry individual policies.

c. Follow-up

Follow-up in this situation can be in two phases, short-term and long-term.

Short-term follow-up could involve the following:

1. Check Mark's immunization records and advise hospital emergency room of the status of his tetanus immunization.
2. Mark has a sister in the school. You should tell her what happened and assure her that her brother will be all right.
3. Explore area of accident on playground to determine what might be done to prevent a recurrence. Safety of the school environment, both interior and exterior, is part of the school nurse's responsibilities. Reassessment of the accident site should occur before making specific recommendations to school officials for increasing safety precautions and preventing future accidents.
4. Make arrangements to inform the other children in the school of Mark's condition. This will give the children an opportunity to ask questions and receive accurate information. Providing children with this opportunity helps to prevent the spread of inaccurate information among the children. Violation of confidentiality must be carefully considered when using this approach. The primary concern is to eliminate inaccurate, inappropriate information.
5. Follow up with Mark and his family to begin planning for continuation of Mark's studies as soon as he is ready, i.e., tutor in hospital, tutor at home, return to school.
6. Plan a conference between Mark, parents, teachers, and school nurse when Mark returns to school to ensure a smooth transition.

The short-term follow-up has focused primarily on the individual client and family. The long term follow-up will expand to include the total population of the school.

The population (aggregate) that the school nurse works with is essentially a well population. A major role of the community health nurse when working with a well population is primary prevention (Spradley, 1985). Shamansky and Clausen (1980, p. 106) define primary prevention as "prevention in the true sense of the word; it precedes disease or dysfunction and is applied to a generally healthy population. The targets are those individuals considered physically or emotionally healthy exhibiting normal or maximal functioning. Primary prevention is not therapeutic; it does not consist of symptom identification and use of therapeutic skills."

There are two categories of primary prevention: (1) specific disease prevention and (2) health promotion. *Health promotion* is described as "generalized and geared to improving people's functioning level in general rather than to ward off or treat a specific disease condition" (Archer & Fleshman, 1979, p. 230). Health promotion is accomplished through health education by teaching people (1) how their habits and life-style influence their health status; (2) how to take responsibility for their choices, and how to effectively take care of themselves (Archer & Fleshman, 1979, p. 230). Health promotion can readily take place within a school setting through health education.

The situation with Mark is an example of how an accident involving one child can have positive long-term effects on the total school population. Such a situation could inspire the school nurse to review how accident prevention is taught within the school. The areas the nurse may look for within the curriculum might include the following:

1. Safety crossing streets
2. Bicycle safety
3. Playground safety (involving playground equipment)
4. Wearing seat belts
5. Preventing athletic injuries with use of appropriate equipment
6. Safety in babysitting
7. Safety in caring for younger brothers and sisters

Yet some may ask: Is accident prevention an appropriate role for the school nurse? For the school? One has only to look at statistics to see the validity of a well-designed accident prevention program. The leading cause of death in American children ages 1 to 14 is accidents. Motor vehicle accidents are responsible for 20 percent of childhood deaths, drownings for 8 percent, and fires for 6 percent (Public Health Service, 1979, p. 39).

Recreational activities and equipment account for the majority of accidents in older children; for example, in 1976:

Age group	Type of accident
6 to 11	Bicycle, swing, skateboard
12 to 17	Football, basketball, bicycle
	(Public Health Service, 1979, p. 39)

Plan for long-term follow-up:

1. Review literature regarding the incidence of accidents in children.
2. Review the roster in the health room, looking specifically for accident-related injuries. (Also keep in mind that many accidents in which children are involved occur away from the school.)
3. Review how the concept of physical safety is approached by teachers in the school, i.e., specific content and at what grade levels.
4. Meet with the principal to discuss your findings and concerns.
5. Discuss your findings and concerns with faculty in a formal faculty meeting.

6. If faculty support your concerns, form a committee of interested individuals to determine how the concept of physical safety could be integrated more effectively into the school curriculum.
7. Discuss the committee's suggestions with the total faculty.
8. Serve as a resource person for teachers as they plan for and integrate safety content into their classrooms (Fredlund, 1967).
9. Evaluate the effectiveness of the new teaching over the next few years.

Resolution

Mark's parents returned home from their trip the following day. In the meantime they were frequently in communication with Mark, the hospital staff, and physicians by telephone.

An accident report was completed by the school nurse and kept on file at the school. A survey of the accident site was made by the nurse, principal, and maintenance man. Recommendations were made for (1) placing a lightweight fence near the top of the embankment as a reminder to students, and (2) establishing a series of "mini sessions" for all grades with the focus on safety on the playground, in the school building, etc.

Mark's leg was placed in traction for approximately three weeks. After discharge he remained at home for approximately one week. He received tutoring throughout his hospital stay and while at home.

Before he returned to school (in a long leg cast) a conference was held with teachers, tutor, nurse, Mark, and his parents to discuss academics, activity level, and safe transportation.

In addition, faculty voted unanimously to integrate content on physical safety in both classroom and after-school activities. A small committee of teachers and the school nurse identified what areas were currently taught and outlined a plan of new content to be introduced. The school nurse served as a resource person to all teachers and assumed teaching responsibility for some aspects of the content within her own health classes.

References

American Academy of Pediatrics (1981). *School health: A guide for professionals.* Evanston, IL: Author.

American Red Cross (1979). *Advanced first aid and emergency care.* (2d ed.) Garden City, NY: Doubleday.

Archer, S. E., & Fleshman, R. P. (1979). *Community health nursing.* (2d ed.) Belmont, CA: Wadsworth.

Fredlund, D. J. (1967). The route to effective school nursing. *Nursing Outlook* 15(8): 24–28.

Long, B. S. (1983). Emergencies and disasters. In W. J. Phipps, B. C. Long, & N. F. Woods (Eds.). *Medical-surgical nursing.* (2d ed.) St. Louis: Mosby.

Pointer, P., & Lancaster, J. (1984). Assertiveness in community health nursing. In M. Stanhope & J. Lancaster (Eds.). *Community health nursing.* St. Louis: Mosby (pp. 824–842).

Public Health Service (1979). Healthy people: The surgeon general's report on health promotion and disease prevention (DHEW Publication No. 79-55071). Washington, DC: U.S. Government Printing Office.

Shamansky, W. L., & Clausen, C. L. (1980). Levels of prevention: Examination of the concept. *Nursing Outlook* 28: 104–108.

Spradley, B. W. (1985). *Community health nursing: Concepts and practice.* (2d ed.) Boston: Little, Brown.

Wold, S. J. (1981). *School nursing: A framework for practice.* St. Louis: Mosby.

═ SITUATION 8 ═
Something's Wrong with Betsy
═ (Self-Paced) ═

SECTION 8.1 —————————————————————————

Today is Wednesday. Mrs. Bean, the third-grade teacher, has asked you to observe in her classroom. In particular she would like you to observe Betsy Stone (an eight-year-old), whose behavior in the classroom has changed over the past few months. Mrs. Bean has said she does not want to give you additional information at this time because it might influence your observation.

In the work space provided:

    a. Based upon the limited information you have, what particular behavioral situations will you want to observe?
    b. What criteria should be used in assessing Betsy's behavior?
    c. Will one observation provide you with enough data to make an accurate assessment?

Student Work Space ——————————————————————

Turn to the following pages to compare your answers.
    a. behavioral situations – p. 103
    b. criteria – p. 103
    c. enough observations? – p. 104

SECTION 8.2

You have completed your classroom observation of Betsy. Mrs. Bean says she will come to your office during her free period to talk with you. You return to your office and review your notes:

> During the majority of the observation Betsy sat quietly at her desk twirling her hair. She frequently looked around the room and out the window. Betsy did not participate in the class discussion.
>
> At one point, in the middle of the class discussion, Betsy stood up and walked around the room with no apparent purpose. Mrs. Bean asked Betsy to return to her desk; Betsy responded, "No! I will not!" When Betsy refused, several children began to giggle and whisper to each other. In apparent response, Betsy slapped one of the children who was giggling. After slapping the girl Betsy did return and sit at her desk. She folded her arms on the desk and put her head down on her arms.

While thinking about the observations, you look out your office window and see the third-graders on the playground. Betsy is not involved in the group activity; she is swinging on a swing alone. After watching for a few minutes, you see two other girls approach Betsy. One of the girls pushes Betsy's swing. In response Betsy stops the swing and chases the two girls.

In the work space provided:

   a. State your assessment.

Student Work Space

Turn to the following page to compare your answer.
a. assessment – p. 104

SECTION 8.3

Later in the day . . .

Betsy's teacher arrives in your office. You ask Mrs. Bean to share her observations and concerns with you.

Mrs. Bean says she is very much concerned about the changes in Betsy's behavior. She states that at the beginning of the school year Betsy was quiet in nature. She played well with other children, she participated readily in classroom activity, and the quality of her work was highly satisfactory. Approximately three months ago Betsy became increasingly quiet and began to participate less often in class. In the past month there has been a substantial decrease in the quality of Betsy's classwork. In addition, Mrs. Bean says the behaviors which occurred in the classroom today, i.e., striking the other child and not responding to teacher requests, have also become more frequent. Despite Betsy's limited participation in school activities, she "hangs around" after school and doesn't seem to want to go home. Mrs. Bean states that each time she has approached Betsy in an attempt to find out what is causing the changes, Betsy responds by saying, "There's nothing wrong."

Mrs. Bean says she recently talked with Betsy's first- and second-grade teachers regarding Betsy's behavior. Both said Betsy was an active, cooperative child in their classrooms. Betsy is an only child, so there are no siblings in other grades for comparison.

Mrs. Bean also says that Betsy's parents have not responded to the school's semi-annual request for parent-teacher conferences. She has tried to contact them on several occasions but has been unsuccessful.

The information Mrs. Bean presents adds to your data base.

In the work space provided, answer the following:

    a. Has your assessment changed? State your rationale.
    b. Would it be appropriate to involve Mrs. Bean in developing a plan for working with Betsy? State your rationale.
    c. State what you would like to have happen with Betsy (client outcomes).
    d. *Briefly* outline a plan to help Betsy reach the outcomes identified. Support the plan with rationale.

Student Work Space

Turn to the following pages to compare your answers.
    a. assessment – p. 105
    b. should Mrs. Bean be involved? – p. 105
    c. client outcomes – p. 105
    d. plan – p. 105

SECTION 8.4

It is now Friday morning. You attempted to contact Betsy's mother by telephone twice yesterday and again this morning. Each attempt has been unsuccessful. Mrs. Bean stops in your office and tells you that she tried unsuccessfully to talk with Betsy yesterday after school. She wants you to know that she will encourage Betsy to come and see you today.

After lunch Betsy arrives in your office. Betsy's skin color is pale, she has dark circles under her eyes, and she looks tired. Betsy's hair is oily and has not been combed. She has on the same dress she wore to school Wednesday and Thursday. You invite her to sit down. She sits quietly for a few seconds looking at the floor. Without raising her eyes she says, "Mrs. Bean wants me to come and see you because she's worried about me."

In the work space provided:

   a. Identify what specific actions you would take in initiating a thera-peutic relationship with an eight-year-old child.
   b. State the rationale supporting your action(s).

Student Work Space

Turn to the following pages to compare your answers.
a. initiating relationship – p. 108
b. rationale – p. 108

SECTION 8.5

During your meeting there is not a great deal of conversation. Betsy does respond to your touch and holds your hand. You acknowledge to Betsy that both you and Mrs. Bean care about her and are concerned about her. After several periods of silence Betsy tells you she is "okay" and doesn't want to talk any more. She says she wants to go back to class.

Before Betsy leaves your office, you tell her that you will be calling her mother to let her know that you and Mrs. Bean are concerned about her. Betsy responds, "Okay, but my parents have gone away today." You phone Betsy's mother but again are unsuccessful in reaching her.

It is now Monday morning. Betsy arrives in your office complaining of a stomach-ache. As she responds to your questions about how long she has had her stomach-ache, what she ate for breakfast, and what she sees as her options for feeling better, you notice that the bottom half of one of Betsy's top teeth (a permanent tooth) is broken off. You ask her how it happened and she responds, "It was an accident. Last night my mother went to grab my arm and her diamond ring hit my tooth and broke it." You ask if she has seen a dentist and Betsy says "No." When you ask if her mother is planning to take her to a dentist, Betsy's response is "I don't know."

In the work space provided:

    a. Identify what actions by the school nurse you think are indicated based upon the interaction with Betsy this morning.

    b. State rationale for your actions.

Student Work Space

Turn to the following pages to compare your answers.
a. actions by the school nurse – p. 109
b. rationale – p. 109

SECTION 8.6

Betsy calls her mother, and in the course of the conversation Mrs. Stone asks to speak to you. She corroborates Betsy's version of the incident. She says she was not aware that Betsy should be seen as soon as possible by a dentist. She says she is too embarrassed to take Betsy to their family dentist because of the nature of the accident. She then says that you can take Betsy to a dentist.

In the work space provided:

    a. What would your response be to Betsy's mother?

    b. Would you transport Betsy to the dentist's office? Support your decision with rationale.

Student Work Space

Turn to the following pages to compare your answers.
a. response to Betsy's mother – p. 110
b. transporting and rationale – p. 111

SECTION 8.7

Mrs. Stone calls their family dentist and he agrees to see Betsy within the hour. Mrs. Stone arrives at school approximately 15 minutes later and takes Betsy to the dentist.

Approximately 1½ hours later you receive a phone call from Betsy's dentist. He says he thinks it was impossible for Betsy to break her tooth as described by Betsy and her mother. The dentist says he is certain this is a child-abuse situation. However, he is reluctant to report it based upon the limited amount of information he has. He says Betsy and Mrs. Stone left his office about 10 minutes ago and should be arriving at school shortly.

Approximately 15 minutes later Mrs. Stone and Betsy arrive in your office. Betsy is holding her mother's hand. Mrs. Stone's eyes are red; obviously she has been crying. Betsy shows you her tooth and says she wants to go back to class. Betsy returns to her classroom.

You ask Mrs. Stone if she would like to talk and she begins to cry. She says she didn't mean to hit Betsy but that everything in her life has been going wrong. She says Mr. Stone has lost his job and has started drinking again; she says her husband drank heavily several years ago (when Betsy was about four years old) but finally managed to stop with the help of Alcoholics Anonymous. She said that was a difficult time for her; she occasionally lost control and hit Betsy then too. Mrs. Stone says she did get help from a social worker then, but this time she thought she could handle the situation herself. She says she's afraid of what will happen if you report her for child abuse.

In the work space provided:

    a. Do you think this situation should be reported? State your rationale.
    b. If yes, to whom would the report be made?
    c. Identify what you think your role(s) is with Mrs. Stone and Betsy—short-term and long-term.
    d. Identify who (if anyone) at your school should be informed of this situation.

Student Work Space

Turn to the following pages to compare your answers.
a. report situation? – p. 111
b. to whom? – p. 114
c. role(s) with Mrs. Stone and Betsy – p. 115
d. who should be informed? – p. 117

ANSWERS TO SECTION 8.1

a and b. Behavioral situations and criteria for assessing Betsy's behavior.

The population the school nurse works with is essentially a well population, so the nurse must have a sound knowledge of growth and development throughout the life span, with an in-depth knowledge of the age group encompassing the majority of his or her clients (Oda, 1979, p. 499).

Obviously, the information the teacher has given you is limited. However, she has asked you to observe *Betsy's behavior* within the *classroom setting*. In the classroom there are predictable behavioral situations which you can observe, i.e., interaction with teacher, interaction with other children, participation in class, etc. (see below).

It may be tempting to compare Betsy's behavior only with the behavior of the other children in the classroom. However, remember that it is within this group of children that Betsy's behavior problems have drawn the teacher's attention, so this comparison may be inadequate. Your comparison will be more accurate if Betsy's behavior is compared to the norm for her age group (Oda, 1979). Keep in mind there is a wide range of norms. It is highly unlikely that any eight-year-old child will meet the description of the norm 100 percent.

Suggested answer:

a. Behavioral situations	b. Criteria for assessing Betsy's behavior should be based on the norms for social development of the eight-year-old.
1. Interaction with teacher	1. Responsive to adults and willing to listen but also has own opinion; begins rebellion. Begins to realize adults are not always right (Whaley & Wong, 1983). Starts to question parents' ideas, values (Dickenson-Hazard, 1984).
2. Interaction with other children	2. Boy/girl relationships are teasing in nature; prefers the company of "best friends" of the same sex (Whaley & Wong, 1983).
3. Involvement in class activity	3. School is a social rather than academic activity to the eight-year-old. Curious and active within the group (Whaley & Wong, 1983). Enjoys clubs, outings, group activity (Dickenson-Hazard, 1984).
4. Attentiveness to tasks	4. Period of extreme curiosity about world and way things work (Whaley & Wong, 1983).
5. Willingness to participate	5. Willing to participate in group activity. The need to belong to the group emerges (Whaley & Wong, 1983). Happy, strong sense of humor (Dickenson-Hazard, 1984).
6. Response to directions	6. May complain about having to do something, expresses own opinion but will respect the request of the adult (Whaley & Wong, 1983).

c. Will one observation provide you with enough data to make an accurate assessment?

If you said that one observation will not provide you with enough data, congratulations! In this situation you have relatively little information, and one classroom observation is unlikely to give you an accurate picture of the child's behavior. It would be wise to make several observations of Betsy in a variety of settings, i.e., the classroom, the playground, the cafeteria, gym class, etc.

ANSWERS TO SECTION 8.2 ――――――――

a. State your assessment.

Child withdrawn, with some episodes of outwardly aggressive behavior; inappropriate for age group.

At this point the only assessment you can make is how Betsy's behavior in the situations you have observed compares with the norm for her age group. To draw any other conclusions would be inappropriate because of the incompleteness of your data base.

To complete your data base, additional data need to be obtained from several sources, e.g., Betsy's classroom teacher; other teachers with whom Betsy has had consistent contact (physical education, music); Betsy's school record; Betsy's parents; and Betsy herself (American Nurses' Association, 1983).

ANSWERS TO SECTION 8.3

a. Has your assessment changed?

If you answered no, your reasoning might be that even though new (additional) information has been obtained, your data base remains incomplete and therefore your assessment should remain unchanged. Unfortunately, this reasoning ignores the significance of the new information.

If you answered yes, your reasoning might be that you do have new (additional) information, i.e., the observations of the classroom teacher, objective evidence that Betsy's classwork has decreased in quality, and some history from other teachers regarding Betsy's behavior in previous years. All of these data indicate there is a *definite change in Betsy's behavior,* and your assessment should reflect this.

Your assessment will be similar to the following:

Child demonstrating behavior changes inappropriate for age group, i.e., withdrawn, some episodes of outwardly aggressive behavior over a period of three months. Data base incomplete.

Be cautious at this point in drawing conclusions about why the change in Betsy's behavior has occurred. Remember, your data base is incomplete, and additional information needs to be obtained before a more comprehensive assessment can be made.

b. Should Mrs. Bean be involved in developing a plan?

By all means Mrs. Bean should be involved in developing a plan for working with Betsy. As the primary adult in the school setting with whom the child has contact, the classroom teacher plays a major role in a child's life. In Betsy's situation *collaboration* with the classroom teacher is indeed appropriate.

Spradley (1985, p. 94) defines collaboration as "working jointly with others in a common endeavor, cooperating as partners." To meet the needs of individual students and/or the school population, the school nurse must develop skill at collaborating with counselors, physicians, dental hygienists, parents, teachers, etc.

c. What would you like to have happen with Betsy?

Your outcomes for Betsy should be similar to the following:

1. Betsy will be able to verbalize how she feels.
2. Betsy will discontinue aggressive behavior with peers.
3. Betsy will resume close relationships with girlfriends.
4. Betsy will participate constructively in classroom activities.
5. Betsy will be able to demonstrate increased quality in classwork.

d. A plan to help Betsy reach the outcomes identified.

The following plan focuses primarily on gathering additional information to complete your data base. It includes both the classroom teacher and the school nurse. If the plan you have written includes the classroom teacher, well done! If it does not, reexamine why.

Plan	*Rationale*
1. Continue to observe Betsy's behavior.	1. The *classroom teacher* will want to continue to observe Betsy's behavior as she has been doing over the previous three months. Additional observations by the school nurse may or may not be necessary; each situation needs to be evaluated individually. For example, you may not be satisfied with the observations you have made, or you may feel that the information you have needs additional validation.
2. Meet with Betsy.	2. At this point it would be wise for the classroom teacher and the school nurse to meet separately with Betsy. The child's comfort level needs to be considered; a joint meeting with both adults could be overwhelming for the child (U.S. Department of Health and Human Services, 1984).
a. Classroom teacher	a. The *classroom teacher* may want to meet with Betsy initially, as she is the adult (in the school) with whom Betsy has the closest contact. The teacher has indicated that previous attempts to talk with Betsy have been unsuccessful. If the teacher experiences the same results, she can let Betsy know that she has discussed her concerns (regarding the changes in Betsy) with the school nurse and that she would like Betsy to meet with the school nurse.
b. School nurse	b. The *school nurse* can use this initial meeting to begin to establish a therapeutic relationship with Betsy. This will also provide the nurse with an opportunity to gather a more comprehensive data base.
3. Establish a time to meet with Betsy's parent(s)/ guardian(s).	3. In many situations encountered by school nurses the nurse cannot effectively work with the child alone as an individual; the total family needs to be involved (Oda, 1979). Betsy's situation warrants involvement of the family unit. In meeting with Betsy's parent(s)/guardian(s), the *school nurse* and the *classroom teacher* can advise them of their concerns and of the changes in Betsy's behavior. In addition, this is an opportunity to obtain additional information from the parent(s)/ guardian(s) to complete the data base and to see if they can be of assistance in identifying the cause(s) of Betsy's behavior changes.

When arranging a meeting with the parent(s)/guardian(s), location of the meeting needs to be considered. The choices are meeting at the school or the family home. A parent conference within the school setting is more common than in the family home. Either location is appropriate, each having distinct advantages and disadvantages as outlined in the following chart.

Parent Conference

At school

Advantages	*Disadvantages*
Efficient use of time by classroom teacher and school nurse	Do not see family interacting as a unit
	Not a natural setting for the parent(s)/guardian(s)
Access to the child's health record and academic record for evidence of changing academic performance	Child is not generally present
	Scheduling may be difficult for the family, i.e., time conflicting with work, etc.

Home visit (Spradley, 1985; Keeling, 1978)

Advantages	*Disadvantages*
Convenient for the family	Less efficient use of time for the school nurse/teacher
Family can be observed as a unit	
Family can be observed interacting within their own environment	
Child is present	
Family may be more comfortable	
Assessment of the family may be more accurate	

4. Consider consulting with school counselor (if that service is available).	4. Based upon the additional information obtained, referral to the school counselor may be appropriate to assist Betsy in reaching the outcomes previously identified.
5. Maintain open communication between classroom teacher, school nurse, and family.	5. Clear communication will facilitate effective collaboration.

ANSWERS TO SECTION 8.4

a. Identify what specific actions you would take to initiate a therapeutic relationship with an eight-year-old child.
b. State the rationale supporting your action(s).

There is no magic formula for establishing a therapeutic relationship with a client, whether a child or an adult. Some nurses are able to do it effectively; others are not. What do those who are effective do? Three things:

1. They care about the client.
2. They understand the impact they can have on a client when they communicate effectively.
3. They use their knowledge of basic communication practices selectively when establishing a nurse-client relationship.

The following actions (all or some) are suggested in attempting to initiate a therapeutic relationship. How they are used and the order in which they are used will naturally vary with each individual nurse.

a. Initiating a therapeutic relationship	*b. Rationale*
1. Provide privacy.	1. Providing privacy, i.e., providing a private space in the health room, conveys to the child that you value and respect what she has to say.
2. Help Betsy feel comfortable.	2. Sit down with the child so you are at the same eye level. Avoid standing and "looking down" at the child. Sit close to the child; avoid having a desk or table between you and the child.
3. Touch Betsy (Stuart & Sundeen, 1983).	3. Touching the child on the shoulder or taking her hand shows that you accept her.
4. Identify the purpose of the meeting (Stuart & Sundeen, 1983).	4. Either participant can identify the purpose of the meeting. In this situation Betsy has told you why she is here. However, that does not mean she fully understands. Help the child express the purpose and clarify as needed. The child should be clear at all times why she is meeting with you.
5. Show respect for Betsy as an individual (Stuart & Sundeen, 1983).	5. Be open and honest. Let the child know that you value her opinion and that you want her to work with you in planning what will happen.
6. Respond with empathy (Stuart & Sundeen, 1983).	6. Placing yourself in the child's "shoes" helps you to understand more completely what she is experiencing.
7. Respond with genuineness (Stuart & Sundeen, 1983).	7. If the child senses you are sincere in your approach to her, she can be free to be open in return.
8. Respond with warmth (Stuart & Sundeen, 1983).	8. Warmth has to be sincere. If it is forced, the child will reestablish distance.

ANSWERS TO SECTION 8.5

a. Identify what actions by the school nurse you think are indicated based upon the interaction with Betsy this morning.
b. State rationale for your actions.

Based upon the interaction with Betsy, the following actions by the nurse are indicated:

a. Actions	*b. Rationale*
1. Resolution of the initial problem which Betsy says brought her to the health office, i.e., her stomachache.	1. The initial problem should not be discounted and needs to be resolved before moving to the more obvious problem of the broken tooth. By working toward resolution of the stomachache, you show the child you are listening to her. Involve the child in resolution of the stomachache (Uttecht, 1983). Resolution may be as simple as needing something to eat.
2. Explain to Betsy that she will need to be seen by a dentist to receive care for her tooth.	2. Clear communication needs to be maintained between you and the child. The child should know what your assessment is and what plan of care you recommend. Maintaining clear communication does several things. It allows the child to: a. experience the respect you have for her. b. continue to trust you. c. anticipate what will happen to her.
3. Explain to Betsy that her mother will need to be contacted so that she will understand what needs to be done and why. She will need to take Betsy to the dentist.	3. Maintain clear communication as described above.
4. Give Betsy the option of deciding whether or not she would like to call her mother.	4. It is tempting to make the decision to call the parent/guardian and then proceed to make the call without involving the child. Whenever possible, the child should be allowed to make the choice.
5. Explain to Betsy that you are willing to talk with her mother regarding your concerns and recommendations.	5. The child should know that you are willing to act as an advocate for her.

a. **Actions**	*b.* **Rationale**
6. Talk to Betsy's mother. Explain to her that you are concerned about Betsy's tooth. Explain to her that in situations where a tooth is broken, dentists want to assess the child's tooth as soon as possible to determine whether the tooth can be preserved. With advanced technology in dental care, many teeth can be saved. When talking with Betsy's mother, two other areas need to be addressed:	6. Remember your primary concern at this time is care of the child and her tooth. The phone call is not necessarily the appropriate time for gathering further data regarding how the situation occurred or for telling the mother how she should have handled the situation. The rationale discussed above (clear communication) applies to the mother as well as the child.
a. Does the family have a dentist or do they need to be referred to one, and	a. The school may have a contractual agreement with a local dentist to provide care to children of families without a family dentist and/or in emergency situations.
b. Are finances a factor in determining whether or not the child will receive care?	b. If finances are a factor, the school nurse usually has knowledge of resources available so that the necessary care can be provided.
7. Follow up with Betsy and her mother.	7. Once the child has received care it would be appropriate to meet with the mother to discuss your concerns regarding the changes in Betsy's behavior, complete your data base, and further assess the total situation.

ANSWERS TO SECTION 8.6 ⸻

a. What would be your response to Betsy's mother?

This is a difficult situation. Your approach to Betsy's mother can have either a positive or negative effect on two things: (1) Betsy's care, and (2) initiating a therapeutic relationship with Betsy's mother.

The actions discussed earlier for initiating a therapeutic relationship with the child (page 108) also apply here in initiating a therapeutic relationship with the child's mother. In addition, the nurse needs to be acutely aware of not allowing personal values to interfere. For example, the situation presented thus far (the various changes in the child's behavior, an incident between parent and child resulting in injury to the child) is one in which the nurse could "jump to conclusions." The nurse can be effective only if personal values are kept in perspective (U.S. Department of Health and Human Services, 1984).

The nurse's initial response is significant, as the mother is already defensive and embarrassed to take Betsy to her dentist because of the nature of the "accident." If the initial response of the nurse is *aggressive,* i.e., threatening, condescending, judgmental, etc., in tone and/or in actual statement, there is a risk the mother will become more defensive, angry, or uncooperative.

If the response of the nurse is accepting of the mother's feelings and nonjudgmental in tone and actual statement, the chances are greater that the mother will listen to what the nurse has to say. Statements like "I can understand this must be difficult" or "I can understand the embarrassment" are *assertive.* They are non-accusatory in nature, they acknowledge how the mother feels, and they give her the opportunity to ventilate her feelings (Pointer & Lancaster, 1984).

Follow up with statements which are *firm, reinforcing* to the mother the need for Betsy to be taken to the dentist; e.g., "It is important for your dentist to assess Betsy's tooth since he knows Betsy and has her dental records. Please call me back after talking with the dentist. I will have Betsy ready to leave school." In the above statements you are giving the responsibility to the mother to follow through with calling the dentist, making an appointment, and transporting her child.

b. Would you transport Betsy to the dentist's office?

If you said you *would not* transport Betsy, good for you! It can be tempting for the school nurse to move into the caretaker role, assuming responsibility for the child and rescuing the mother from an unpleasant situation. Is that the role of the school nurse? Isn't the more appropriate role one in which the nurse assists the mother in dealing with an uncomfortable situation and taking responsibility for her own child?

Oda (1979) states that "the main focus in school nursing regardless of age, grade, or other characteristics of the client population is on what can be called *educational health*—that is, those aspects of health that influence the individual student's or the group's learning ability." Obviously whatever is happening in Betsy's life is affecting her learning ability. The school nurse needs to be involved with this child and her family, but transporting Betsy to and from the dentist is not the best way of fulfilling that role.

Some may argue that in some situations it would be to the child's advantage if the nurse did assume a caretaker role. *Each situation needs to be evaluated carefully before the nurse makes a decision*; e.g., in an acute emergency situation, transportation by the nurse may indeed be appropriate. In each school/school district there are generally guidelines outlining when it is and when it is not appropriate to transport children. A pragmatic concern of the school district is liability for the child should an accident occur while a child is being transported by a staff member.

ANSWERS TO SECTION 8.7

a. Do you think this situation should be reported?

If you think this situation should be reported, you are correct. Remember, abused children cannot receive protection unless they are identified. From 1963 to 1968 all states mandated that cases of *suspected* child abuse and neglect must be reported by health professionals (Wold, 1981). In recent years most states have expanded their laws, requiring teachers and school personnel as well as health professionals to report suspected child abuse.

State statutes vary, but all contain some common elements: i.e., a definition of child abuse and neglect, who must report, to whom the report is made, and the content of the report. No state requires that the individual making the report have proof that abuse has occurred. The report can be based on suspected incidents (U.S. Department of Health and Human Services, 1984). The enactment of reporting laws in all fifty of the United States has raised the possibility that courts could label failure to report·child abuse as negligence *per se* in malpractice litigation (Bross, 1983, p. 71). Because of the differences from state to state, school nurses and educators should review their state's child abuse and neglect law. *This is a good time for you as nursing students to review the laws on child abuse in your state.*

Each school district should also have policies which correspond to the state statutes and outline in detail the responsibilities of the school and its professionals. Individual school policies may provide specific guidelines such as:

1. Who actually makes the report, i.e., school nurse, teacher, principal.
2. How involved the individual making the report should become with the child's family.
3. Procedures for documentation (U.S. Department of Health and Human Services, 1984).

What constitutes child abuse?

Child abuse can be divided into four main categories: physical abuse, physical neglect, sexual abuse, and emotional abuse and neglect. They are defined as follows:

Wold (1981) describes *physical abuse* as active abuse causing injury to the child by another person irrespective of the age of the abuser. Physical abuse can be the result of one or repeated episodes. The intensity of the abuse can range from mild (bruises) to severe (fractures, internal injuries), in some situations causing death. The types of *injuries most often seen in the school-age child* involve soft tissue damage such as abrasions, lacerations, swelling, welts, and burns. More serious injuries and even death can result from physical abuse in younger children as the younger child cannot fight back or flee from the abuser. In physical-abuse situations the description of the accident is often not consistent with the type of injury the child has sustained.

Physical neglect is best described as failure on the part of the parent(s)/guardian(s) to meet the basic physiological needs of the child, i.e., food, clothing, shelter, and access to medical care (Wold, 1981; Nix, 1980).

Sexual abuse can be described as contacts or interactions between a child and an adult in which the child is used for sexual purposes by the adult, or the adult is the intermediary providing the child to be used for sexual purposes by another adult (Nix, 1980; U.S. Department of Health and Human Services, 1984).

Emotional abuse and neglect is not easily defined. Wold (1981) describes it as a rejection by the parent(s)/guardian(s)—rejection that attacks the child's self-esteem and sense of self-worth.

How is the abused child recognized?

Abused children present with a wide range of physical and behavioral indicators. The following are some of those indicators:

Type of abuse	Physical indicators	Behavioral indicators
Physical abuse	Unexplained bruises and welts Unexplained burns Unexplained fractures Unexplained lacerations Unexplained abdominal injuries Human bite marks Sudden or insidious appearance of a combination of above injuries	Is wary of contact with adults (pulls away from physical closeness with adults) Is apprehensive when other children cry Displays extremes in behavior, i.e., withdrawn to aggressive Is frightened of parents Does not want to go home Reports an injury by the parent

(U.S. Department of Health and Human Services, 1984, pp. 14–16; Lancaster & Kerschner, 1984)

Type of abuse	Physical indicators	Behavioral indicators
Physical neglect	Constant hunger, poor hygiene Inappropriate clothing Consistent lack of supervision Constant fatigue or listlessness Unattended physical problems or medical needs Abandonment	Begs or steals food Constantly falls asleep in class Rarely attends school Comes to school very early, leaves very late Is addicted to drugs or alcohol Engages in delinquent activities States that there is no one to care for him or her

(U.S. Department of Health and Human Services, 1984, pp. 16–17)

Type of abuse	Physical indicators	Behavioral indicators
Sexual abuse	Difficulty sitting or walking Torn, stained, or bloody underclothing Complaints of pain or itching in the genital area Bruises or bleeding in external genitalia, vaginal area, or anal area Sexually transmitted disease (especially in a child under 13) Pregnancy, especially in early adolescence	Appears withdrawn, engages in fantasy, may even appear retarded Has poor peer relationships Is unwilling to change clothes for gym or participate in physical activities Engages in delinquent acts Runs away Displays bizarre, sophisticated, or unusual sexual knowledge or behavior Reports sexual assault by a caretaker

(U.S. Department of Health and Human Services, 1984, p. 18)

Type of abuse	Physical indicators	Behavioral indicators
Emotional abuse and neglect		Habit disorders, i.e., sucking, rocking, biting, feeding disorders
		Conduct disorders, i.e., withdrawal, antisocial behavior
		Neurotic traits, i.e., sleep disorders, inhibition of play
		Psychoneurotic reactions, i.e., hysteria, obsession, compulsion, hypochondria
		Behavior extremes, i.e., passive to aggressive
		Overly adaptive behaviors, i.e., parenting other children or acting extremely infantile
		Lag in emotional development
		Attempted suicide or conversations about suicide

(Wald, 1961, pp. 6–7)

b. To whom would the report be made?

In each state, a specific state agency is identified to receive reports of child abuse. The appointed agency is usually the department of public welfare, social services, or human resources. Other agencies which may be required by law to receive reports of child abuse are the police department, health department, juvenile or district court, or county or district attorney's office (U.S. Department of Health and Human Services, 1984, p. 33).

The process of reporting a suspected child-abuse situation should be kept uncomplicated but should include the following:

1. Child's name and address
2. Parent(s)/guardian(s) name and address
3. Child's date of birth
4. Name of child's teacher and grade level
5. Date of the report
6. Name and title of the individual filing the report
7. Telephone number of the individual filing the report
8. A description of the injury/condition
9. The basis for the belief abuse exists
(Wold, 1981)

There may be a time frame for filing a report of suspected child abuse, i.e., 24-48 hours from the time an incident is identified. If a time frame is specified, it will be defined in the state statute.

The school nurse may be a valuable resource to the agency (department of public welfare, etc.) on following up on the child-abuse report. However, the school nurse must remain cognizant of the rights of the child and parent/guardian regarding confidentiality and may share information only with those individuals identified by state law (U.S. Department of Health and Human Services, 1984).

Documentation by the school nurse of the incident(s) that led to the reporting of suspected child abuse or neglect is essential. Documentation needs to comply with policies established by the local school district and the state law. However, the following criteria should be met:

1. Documentation begins at the *onset* of eacn suspected incident.
2. Observations are presented in an objective manner.
3. Subjectivity by the nurse is avoided.

(Kreitzer, 1981)

c. Identify your roles with Mrs. Stone and Betsy—short-term and long-term.

Short-term roles with Mrs. Stone

Provider of care. At this moment, Mrs. Stone is experiencing an acute crisis. The nurse needs to remain in a therapeutic role. By doing so, the nurse allows Mrs. Stone the freedom to ventilate her feelings and identify her frustrations, fears, and concerns. The nursing actions for establishing a therapeutic relationship certainly apply, i.e., touch, eye contact, respect, genuineness, empathy, etc. These practices can be reviewed on page 108.

Once again, the nursing process provides the framework for intervention with Mrs. Stone (Stuart & Sundeen, 1983, pp. 629–634):

Assessment:	Determining what has precipitated the crisis. Helping the client identify her strengths and coping mechanisms. Helping the client identify the nature and strength of her support systems.
Planning:	Exploring the client's options and the specific steps to reach a solution.
Intervention:	Intervention can occur in several ways. A school nurse who has expertise in counseling clients may choose to begin counseling Mrs. Stone on a one-to-one basis. Other school nurses may choose to provide Mrs. Stone with general support and *refer* her to the community resource which will benefit her the most, i.e., the school counselor, a community counselor, social worker, department of public welfare, community self-help groups.
Evaluation:	Reviewing the acute situation and determining both client and nurse satisfaction with the resolution.

Referrer. There are a variety of community agencies to which the school nurse can refer Mrs. Stone as mentioned above. A more complete description will be presented under the long-term roles.

Short-term role with Betsy

Referrer. Referral of Betsy, with her mother's knowledge and permission, to the school counselor (if the school provides that service) is indeed appropriate.

Betsy has been experiencing abusive behavior from her mother, but she is also witnessing alcohol abuse by her father. Triplett and Arbeson (1983, p. 318) identify the following as needs of children from alcoholic/abusive families:

1. Establishing and maintaining a primary relationship with an adult.
2. Learning about alcoholism as a disease.
3. Acknowledging that a parent is an alcoholic.
4. Knowing when and how to get help.
5. Learning to feel worthwhile.

The school nurse can advise Betsy's mother of the counseling services available to her child and the appropriateness of using the service.

Long-term roles with Mrs. Stone

Referrer. Referring Mrs. Stone to community resources is an appropriate role for the school nurse. The following resources are appropriate for referral:

1. The social worker from the department of public welfare with whom Mrs. Stone worked several years ago.
2. The school counselor (if that service is available) for family counseling or at least counseling for Mrs. Stone and Betsy.
3. A community-based counselor if one is not available through the school.
4. Al-Anon – a self-help group for families who have an alcoholic member.
5. Alcoholics Anonymous – a self-help group for the individual who has a problem with alcohol.
6. Parents Anonymous – a self-help group for parents who have abused their children.

The concept of self-help groups unfortunately is still foreign to many health care professionals. The focus of the self-help group is one of people helping people gain and maintain control over the problems in their lives. Within the group, the individual has a chance to discuss fears, frustrations, etc., with others who can genuinely empathize because they have been confronted with similar problems in their own lives. Participation in the group brings about a new sense of awareness and improved self-esteem. Positive reinforcement from the group is another benefit. With time, the individual develops a new sense of responsibility for personal behavior (Nix, 1980).

Self-help groups are increasing in number throughout the country. Alcoholics Anonymous, Al-Anon, Overeaters Anonymous, Gamblers Anonymous, and Parents Anonymous are some of the more widely publicized groups.

If you have never attended a self-help group meeting to understand what happens there, perhaps you should.

Advocate. The school nurse may serve as an advocate for the child with teachers and parents, or for the total family unit with department of public welfare, juvenile court, etc., should the need arise.

Consultant. The family may use the nurse as a consultant regarding appropriate use of community resources, i.e., counseling, department of public welfare.

Long-term roles with Betsy

Provider of care. In the future Betsy may (or may not) seek assistance/support from the school nurse as her family situation becomes more positive, remains unchanged, or becomes more stressed.

Referrer. The rationale discussed under short-term roles also applies. In addition, if the quality of Betsy's classwork does not improve, the school nurse may *collaborate* with the classroom teacher and refer Betsy for special education services. Public Law 94-142, the Education for All Handicapped Children Act of 1975, mandates that children who have special needs should have an individualized educational plan (I.E.P.) developed for them.

d. Identify who (if anyone) at your school should be informed of this situation.

1. *Principal.* The principal has a responsibility to the community to see that children attending the school are receiving appropriate services. In some schools the principal assumes the role of spokesperson in reporting child-abuse situations to the department of public welfare.
2. *Classroom teacher.* For the past several months the teacher has been attempting to understand the changes she has observed in Betsy. With this new information she will be better equipped to work with Betsy within the classroom setting. She will be able to monitor Betsy's behavior changes, both positive or negative, and to plan early intervention and/or consultation with the nurse or counselor if negative behavior patterns recur.
3. *Counselor.* The counselor can provide Betsy and her parents with the appropriate guidance to assist them in resolving or adapting to the stress-producing situations in their lives.

Resolution

The school nurse did contact the department of public welfare to report the child-abuse situation, and Mrs. Stone was put in contact with the social worker she had seen previously. Both Betsy and Mrs. Stone are receiving counseling through the school guidance department. The physical abuse has stopped and Betsy's aggressive behavior at school has subsided. Betsy's level of activity and attentiveness at school have increased. She has become actively involved in group play and is spending individual time with two other girls in her class. Mrs. Stone is attending a weekly Al-Anon meeting and finding it beneficial in helping her deal with her husband's alcohol problem. Mrs. Stone has been introduced to the Parents Anonymous group, but at this time is not attending meetings. Betsy's father remains unemployed but has started attending Alcoholics Anonymous meetings several times a week. He has recently expressed an interest in participating in the counseling sessions with Betsy and his wife.

In this situation with the Stone family, the resolution has been positive, with both parents willing to accept responsibility for their behavior. Unfortunately, this does not always happen, and the pattern as described in this situation often repeats itself.

References

American Nurses' Association (1983). *Standards of school nursing practice* (NP-66 5M 7/83). Kansas City, MO: Author.

Bross, D. (1983). Professional and agency liability for negligence in child protection. *Law, Medicine and Health Care* 11(2):71–75.

Dickenson-Hazard, N. (1984). School age children and adolescents. In M. Stanhope & J. Lancaster (Eds.). *Community health nursing.* St. Louis: Mosby (pp. 581–620).

Keeling, B. L. (1978). Making the most of the first home visit. *Nursing '78* 8(24):24–28.

Kreitzer, M. (1981). Legal aspects of child abuse. *Nursing Clinics of North America* 16(1):149–160.

Lancaster, J., & Kerschner, D. (1984). Violence and human abuse as community health problems. In M. Stanhope & J. Lancaster (Eds.). *Community health nursing.* St. Louis: Mosby (pp. 446–464).

Nix, H. (1980). Why parents anonymous? *Journal of Psychiatric Nursing and Mental Health Services* 18: 23–28.

Oda, D. (1979). Community nursing in schools: Developing a specialized role. In S. E. Archer & R. P. Fleshman (Eds.). *Community health nursing.* (2d ed.) Belmont, CA: Wadsworth (pp. 495–510).

Pointer, P., & Lancaster, J. (1984). Assertiveness in community health nursing. In M. Stanhope & J. Lancaster (Eds.). *Community health nursing.* St. Louis: Mosby (pp. 824–842).

Spradley, B. W. (1985). *Community health nursing: Concepts and practice.* (2d ed.) Boston: Little, Brown.

Stuart, G. W., & Sundeen, S. J. (1983). *Principles and practice of psychiatric nursing.* (2d ed.) St. Louis: Mosby.

Triplett, J. L., & Arbeson, S. W. (1983). Working with children of alcoholics. *Pediatric Nursing* 9(5):317–320.

U.S. Department of Health and Human Services (1984). *The educator's role in the prevention and treatment of child abuse and neglect* (HEW-105-77-1050). Washington, DC: Author.

Uttecht, J. (1983). Teaching children responsibility for health. *Vermont Registered Nurse,* January 1983, 5–6.

Wald, M. (1961). *Protective services and emotional neglect.* Denver: The American Humane Association.

Whaley, L. F., & Wong, D. L. (1983). *Nursing care of infants and children.* St. Louis: Mosby.

Wold, S. (1981). *School nursing: A framework for practice.* St. Louis: Mosby.

PART III

Maternal-Child Health

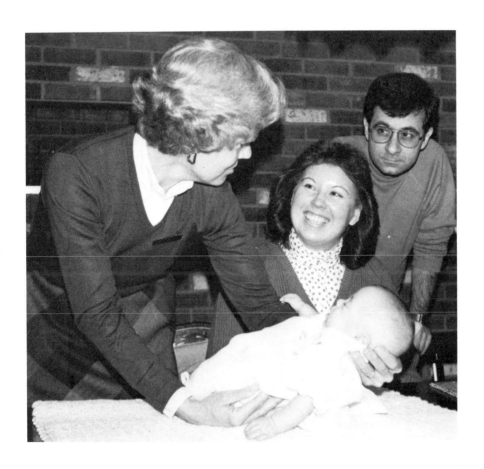

SITUATION 9
More to Do Than Meets the Eye
(Self-Paced)

SECTION 9.1

You are a staff nurse employed by Stanton County Health Services. Maternal-child health is the primary focus of this official agency.

A nurse with whom you work will be going on a maternity leave. On recommendation of the supervisor she is turning management of a few of her clients over to you. Some of these clients are high-risk pregnant women with well-defined medical problems, and some are described as normal. One is Mrs. Williams, a 28-year-old primigravida. She is in her third trimester, healthy, a college graduate, with a sound, financially stable marriage. She was last seen by the nurse three weeks ago, at which time she seemed apprehensive about labor and delivery and initial care of the baby.

As the nurse is describing Mrs. Williams to you, she says that since Mrs. Williams is basically "doing well" and is attending expectant parent classes, you probably will not need to see her until she has had her baby. Her due date is four weeks away.

In the work space provided answer the following questions:

    a. Do you agree with the nurse? Assuming your time commitments permit, would you see Mrs. Williams again before delivery? Support your decision with rationale. If you decided not to see her, stop here.

    b. If you would see her, what would be the focus of your visits? Support your answer with rationale.

    c. What level of prevention would you be practicing—primary, secondary, or tertiary? Why?

Student Work Space

Turn to the following pages to compare your answers.
    a. would you see Mrs. Williams? – p. 124
    b. focus of visits – p. 125
    c. level of prevention – p. 127

121

SECTION 9.2

In thinking about Mrs. Williams in her third trimester, you could expect that she may be experiencing some or all of the body changes listed below.

In the work space provided:

    a. Identify the causes of the body changes.
    b. Briefly identify what nursing actions/interventions would be appropriate.

Student Work Space

Body changes	Cause(s)	Nursing actions/ interventions
1. Heartburn		
2. Frequent urination		
3. Edema		
4. Leg cramps		
5. Varicose veins		
6. Constipation		
7. Hemorrhoids		
8. Backache		

Turn to the following pages to compare your answers.
a. causes – p. 127
b. nursing interventions – p. 127

SECTION 9.3

Within the next week, you telephone Mrs. Williams and arrange a time for a home visit. When you arrive at the Williamses' home, you spend time assessing Mrs. Williams's progress in her third trimester. She says she has been preparing for the baby's arrival; the baby's room is almost ready and she has only a few items left to buy. She says that she and her husband have started attending expectant parent classes. However, she has some concerns that have not been addressed in the classes. She gives you the following information:

> "I had a friend who was admitted to the hospital twice in false labor. I don't want that to happen to me. How am I going to know the difference between false labor and real labor?"

> "I am scared about the pain I'll have during labor. Is there anything I can do to help prepare myself?"

> "I have decided I'd like to try breastfeeding. Is it too late to make that decision? What can I do to get ready?"

In the work space provided, answer the following questions:

a. What would you *say* in your *initial response* to Mrs. Williams? (Write your exact words.)
b. What do you want your initial response to *convey* to Mrs. Williams and why?
c. A major nursing intervention at this time is client education. Outline below what you would teach Mrs. Williams based upon her questions. Include rationale.

Student Work Space

(continued)

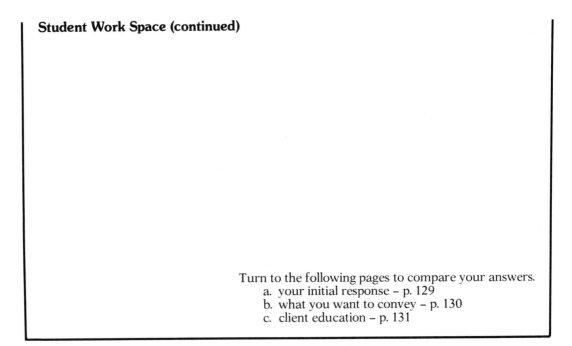

Student Work Space (continued)

Turn to the following pages to compare your answers.
a. your initial response – p. 129
b. what you want to convey – p. 130
c. client education – p. 131

ANSWERS TO SECTION 9.1

a. Would you see Mrs. Williams again before delivery?

This is a situation in which there may be a significant amount of disagreement. If you agree with the nurse that it is not necessary to see Mrs. Williams, your rationale may be similar to that of the nurse—i.e., since the client is healthy, has no complications, and is managing well on her own, you think your nursing knowledge can be more effectively used with the high-risk pregnant clients.

Some of you may have pointed out that the size of your workload (caseload) would have a bearing on your decision. Your reasoning here may be that if the caseload is heavy, with a large number of multiproblem clients, you will want to use your time where you think you can have the greatest impact—with the high-risk pregnant women, leaving those who are well to care for themselves.

There is a tendency among health professionals to limit their therapeutic role to clients/families with well-defined problems. Such a philosophy perpetuates the "fire fighting" approach and neglects the professional nurse's major role through anticipatory guidance. Is there a clue for therapeutic intervention by the nurse in Mrs. Williams's apprehension about labor and delivery as well as initial care of the baby? Giving her more information and discussing her worries with her might well make the difference between an anxious client and a client who approaches with confidence not only labor and delivery but also the early days of caring for the new baby at home.

The results of working with the well pregnant woman and her family are not as easily identified and measured as they are with the high-risk client. It may also seem less exciting to help a well pregnant woman progress through pregnancy, labor, delivery, and the transition to home without complications or stress than to work with a high-risk client—for example, a pregnant adolescent who, through counseling by the community health nurse on proper diet and smoking cessation during pregnancy, delivers a normal, healthy, full-term infant.

There is no question that high-risk pregnant women *are* indeed a priority when determining which clients to visit. Unfortunately, when funding puts constraints on the number of staff available, the needs of the "well" expectant family are neglected, and unnecessary problems develop. In an adequately funded program, nurses who reason that the high-risk pregnant women are their only priority will find themselves with a skewed caseload. A caseload of high-risk multiproblem pregnant women and families can be frustrating for the nurse. In a caseload consisting only of high-risk pregnant women, the nurse must concentrate on *solving problems*—i.e., "fire fighting"—and has little time to devote to *preventing problems* through anticipatory guidance.

With a caseload balanced between well pregnant women and high-risk pregnant women the nurse experiences the benefits of both anticipatory guidance and problem solving. The satisfactions derived from working with healthy mothers and babies provide the nurse with renewed energy for effective problem solving with the high-risk pregnant woman.

If your decision was not to see Mrs. Williams, did you think you had sufficient data on which to base your decision? The client has not been seen by the nurse for three weeks, during which time changes could have occurred. A telephone call to Mrs. Williams would be appropriate at this time to allow you to gather additional data before making a decision. In addition, the telephone call provides you with an opportunity to introduce yourself to the client, and it is a means of notifying the client of your plans regarding her care and follow-up.

If you do not agree with the nurse and indicated you would see Mrs. Williams, your supporting rationale should be based on the premise that the nurse can play a meaningful role with the well pregnant woman and her family as well as with the high-risk pregnant woman and her family.

b. Focus of visits

The focus of visits to this healthy primigravida can consist of two major concepts, *health promotion* and *anticipatory guidance* (Tegtmeier & Elsea, 1984). Both of these concepts are appropriate for community health nurses to integrate into their practice when working with healthy clients and/or groups. Health promotion and anticipatory guidance are concepts that are not completely understood by many nurses and health care professionals in general.

Health promotion is described as "generalized and geared to improving people's functioning level in general rather than to ward off or treat a specific disease condition" (Archer & Fleshman, 1979, p. 230). Health promotion is accomplished through health education by teaching people (1) how their habits and life-style influence their health status; (2) how to take responsibility for their choices and how to effectively take care of themselves (Archer & Fleshman, 1979, p. 230).

When working with the pregnant woman, the nurse has an opportunity to assist the client in maintaining her own level of wellness during pregnancy and in providing a healthy environment for her unborn child through teaching on pregnancy, nutrition, exercise, rest, stress management, and avoidance of chemical abuse, i.e., smoking, alcohol, medications.

At present, the major focus of the health care system in the United States is care and cure of disease. Very little emphasis is placed on health promotion. People have difficulty seeing benefits to health promotion, as results occur slowly over a long period of time and are not easily measured. People have less difficulty understanding care/cure of a disease process, as results are readily observable and, therefore, measurable.

Anticipatory guidance as described by Elkins (1984) is the ability to anticipate maturational and situational events which are stress producing and have crisis potential, and then working with the individual and family to help them through the developmental phase. Teaching clients what to anticipate as they move through the life process and helping them identify resources and sources of strength can help them adapt to and cope with a situation more effectively.

Maturational events (Elkins, 1984, p. 290) requiring anticipatory guidance can be characterized as events related to normal growth and development; i.e., pregnancy, the expanding family, childhood development, adolescence, young adulthood, and marriage. Progression through these life processes can be stress producing and in some individuals and families can result in crises. Hymovich (1979, p. 32) states, "The purpose of anticipatory guidance for expectant parents is to meet their informational needs before they arise, thereby diminishing anxiety, trauma, and the possibility of compounded crises before they occur."

Situational events (Elkins, 1984, p. 290) requiring anticipatory guidance can be characterized as unexpected events that occur in the life process, e.g., illness (physical or mental), divorce, accidents, death of a friend or family member, or loss of employment. Anticipatory guidance in both maturational and situational events allows the client/family to see that they are not alone in what they are experiencing, that their concerns are valid, and that effective ways of coping with their stress do exist.

Anticipatory guidance is an integral part of the nurse's role with Mrs. Williams. Pregnancy is generally a normal life process for an individual and her family. The following developmental stages are involved (Olds, London, & Ladewig, 1984):

1. The married couple – prior to pregnancy, establishing themselves as a couple, establishing a home, developing a life-style as a couple, etc.
2. The beginning family phase – deciding on pregnancy, adapting to (accepting) the pregnancy as a couple, adapting to sexual patterns, future planning regarding finances, establishing work responsibilities. During this period the pregnant woman is also experiencing physiological changes related to the pregnancy.
3. Child-rearing family period – adapting to a new person in the family, reestablishing satisfying sexual patterns, making adaptations in work distribution.

Each of the above periods can be stress producing for the family. Through the use of anticipatory guidance by the community health nurse, however, the stress can be minimized or avoided altogether.

A third concept that may be difficult for nurses and health care professionals to understand is the *well family.* "The well family is a dynamic unit whose members are engaged in tasks aimed at both personal development and continuation of the family system. Furthermore, the family is a social unit representing traditions; special communication patterns; a life history of experiences, beliefs, values, and norms; and interpersonal competencies that enable the members to interact with society and one another, achieve goals, and fulfill dreams" (Petze, 1984, p. 234). The role of the nurse with the well family is to assist the family, as individuals and as a unit, to achieve an optimum level of functioning. This is accomplished through health promotion and anticipatory guidance.

c. Level of prevention

The level of prevention practiced in this situation is without a doubt *primary prevention.* Shamansky and Clausen (1980, p. 106) define primary prevention as "prevention in the true sense of the word; it precedes disease or dysfunction and is applied to a generally healthy population. The targets are those individuals considered physically or emotionally healthy exhibiting normal or maximal functioning. Primary prevention is not therapeutic; it does not consist of symptom identification and use of therapeutic skills."

Health promotion and anticipatory guidance are the essence of primary prevention. The healthy pregnant client probably offers one of the best opportunities for the community health nurse to practice primary prevention. The nurse can assist the pregnant woman in maintaining and improving her own level of wellness and at the same time is working with the pregnant woman to produce a healthy new individual.

ANSWERS TO SECTION 9.2

a and b. Causes and nursing actions/interventions

Body changes	a. Cause(s) (Bobak & Jensen, 1984; Olds et al., 1984)	b. Nursing actions/ interventions (Bobak & Jensen, 1984; Olds et al., 1984)
1. Heartburn (pyrosis)	Increasing size of the uterus causes displacement of the stomach and relaxation of the cardiac sphincter, leading to regurgitation of gastric juices; gastic juices cause a burning sensation in the esophagus.	*Client education*: Avoid fatty foods, overeating; take small, frequent meals; wait an hour before lying down after a meal. Avoid use of sodium bicarbonate as it can lead to electrolyte imbalance. Encourage client to choose bland foods.
2. Frequent urination	Increased pressure on the bladder from the enlarging uterus; coughing, sneezing can result in leakage.	*Client education*: Watch for signs/symptoms of urinary tract infection, i.e., burning, itching, fever; maintain fluid intake; practice Kegel exercises (tightening perineal muscles to maintain muscle tone and decrease potential for leakage).
3. Edema	Increased size of the abdomen causes increased pressure on the lower abdomen and groin, thus decreasing	*Client education*: Avoid standing, sitting for prolonged periods of time; avoid constricting stockings, garters; elevate legs during rest periods. Ex-

Body changes	*a. Cause(s)* (Bobak & Jensen, 1984; Olds et al., 1984)	*b. Nursing actions/ interventions* (Bobak & Jensen, 1984; Olds et al., 1984)
	the efficiency of venous return from the lower extremities.	cessive edema in combination with headaches or seeing spots before eyes should be brought to the attention of the obstetrician immediately.
4. Leg cramps	Increased weight of uterus on nerves to the legs; increased weight also decreases efficiency of peripheral circulation; some data would indicate calcium imbalance.	*Client education*: Muscle stretching—teach how to do with/without assistance from another person. May need to have client decrease milk consumption (do not eliminate completely). Encourage client to discuss amount of milk consumption with physician.
5. Varicose veins	Increased weight of the uterus increases pressure on leg veins, thus decreasing efficiency of venous return. The increased pressure also weakens the valves in the leg veins, causing stasis of blood and gradual weakening of the walls of the veins, producing varicosities. (Some women may be predisposed to varicosities by family history.)	*Client education*: Avoid standing, sitting for prolonged periods of time; avoid constricting clothing, i.e., stockings, garters. Encourage use of support hose. Encourage elevation of legs whenever sitting; also encourage lying down on a bed, sofa, floor, etc., at regular times each day, elevating legs above body to facilitate venous return.
6. Constipation	Increased size of uterus displaces intestines, decreasing motility; oral iron supplements may contribute to the problem. (In some women with a predisposition to bowel problems, they will be exaggerated.)	*Client education*: Maintain/ increase fluid intake; encourage fiber/bulk in daily diet. Use of natural bulk, i.e., fruits/vegetables, bran, prune juice preferred to laxatives.

Body changes	a. Cause(s) (Bobak & Jensen, 1984; Olds et al., 1984)	b. Nursing actions/ interventions (Bobak & Jensen, 1984; Olds et al., 1984)
7. Hemor- rhoids	Increased weight of the uterus in- creases pressure on veins around the rectum, weak- ening their walls and producing var- icosities (hemor- rhoids). Women who have diffi- culty with consti- pation may also be increasing pres- sure on the veins by extensive push- ing at the time of bowel movements.	*Client education*: Same as above for avoiding con- stipation. To help de- crease burning, itching, discomfort, teach client how to provide symptom- atic relief from the hemorrhoids—i.e., rein- sertion of the hemor- rhoids (have client lie on her side and, using a lubri- cant, reinsert with fin- ger), warm soaks, ice packs, and topical appli- cations.
8. Back- ache	Increased size and weight of the uter- us cause stretch- ing of the abdom- inal muscles, causing anterior portion of pelvis to tilt forward, thus exaggerating the curvature in the lumbosacral area. Backache may also be caused by the increased size of the breasts if they are not being supported appro- priately.	*Client education*: Avoid lifting, bending; use ap- propriate body mechan- ics. Teach client how to do pelvic tilt exercises— i.e., lie on floor or stand against a wall, bend knees and press curva- ture of lumbosacral area flat to floor or wall. En- courage client to wear a properly fitting brassiere (see p. 132).

ANSWERS TO SECTION 9.3

a. Your initial response.

Your initial response to Mrs. Williams could be similar to one (or a combination) of the following:

> "It sounds as though you have several areas of concern. Would you like to discuss each one separately? I can work with you to . . ."

> "I can understand that the areas you've identified are of con- cern to you. Perhaps through discussion of each area, some of those concerns can be alleviated."

"From the questions you're asking, it sounds as though you've done a lot of thinking and have identified specific areas of concern. Perhaps by addressing each area . . ."

"I understand your concerns. Other pregnant women I work with have identified similar areas of concern. Perhaps by discussing each area I can help alleviate . . ."

b. What you want to convey to Mrs. Williams.

Your initial response to Mrs. Williams needs to be one that will facilitate effective communication between nurse and client. The initial response needs to convey:

1. *Acknowledgment* of the client's concerns
2. *Respect* for the client (Stuart & Sundeen, 1983)
3. *Empathy* regarding the client's concerns (Stuart & Sundeen, 1983)
4. *Reassurance* that the client's concerns can and will be addressed

Acknowledgment of the client's concerns conveys to the client that the nurse is really listening to what the client is saying. Through the use of anticipatory guidance, the nurse can convey to the client that her concerns are valid, justified, and commonly expressed by other pregnant women. Acknowledgment by the nurse needs to be accepting and nonjudgmental in nature. For example, Mrs. Williams will continue to voice her concerns to the nurse if she feels the nurse views her concerns as valid. However, if the nurse pays little attention to what Mrs. Williams says or dismisses the concerns as insignificant, Mrs. Williams may feel inhibited and not discuss further concerns with the nurse.

Respect (Stuart & Sundeen, 1983) – valuing the client and her beliefs. Although the client's values, culture, concerns, and plans may vary substantially from those of the nurse, they are valid. A nurse who disregards a client's values, culture, concerns, plans, etc., is communicating to the client that what she thinks and feels is not important. The nurse can demonstrate respect for Mrs. Williams by remaining nonjudgmental in reacting to her questions and providing her with the information she needs.

Empathy (Stuart & Sundeen, 1983) – allowing oneself to feel what the client is feeling. Realistically, an individual nurse may not be able to feel what each client is feeling through direct experience. However, the nurse may have had an experience that produced very similar feelings. For example, a nurse who has never been through labor and delivery can still empathize with Mrs. Williams's fear of the pain because of a similar personal experience with surgery.

Reassurance that the client's concerns can and will be addressed can be beneficial in reducing stress in the client. Reassurance should be sincere and genuine, not patronizing in nature. The nurse's reassurance should help Mrs. Williams feel more positive and less anxious.

Look back at what you have written as your initial response to Mrs. Williams's concerns. Does your answer convey acknowledgment, respect, empathy, and reassurance? If it does, congratulations! If it doesn't, what's missing? How can you make your response more effective?

c. **Client education – content for teaching**.

Differences between false labor and true labor

Characteristics	False labor	True labor
Frequency of contractions	Generally irregular (Braxton Hicks contractions which may have been occurring at intervals since the fourth month of pregnancy)	Will become regular and increase in frequency
Duration/ intensity of contractions	Generally will not increase	Will increase with frequency
Location of discomfort	Generally lower abdomen and groin area	Back and total abdomen
Alleviation of discomfort	Generally with ambulation and with sedation	Will continue to increase and will intensify with ambulation

(Bobak & Jensen, 1984; Olds et al., 1984)

Although differences in false labor and true labor can be identified, clients should be taught that *often it is impossible to differentiate between the two without a vaginal examination by a physician or nurse midwife in the hospital.* Going to the hospital only to find that one is in false labor may be embarrassing to some clients, but it is far better to err on the side of safety than to risk an unattended birth. (Bobak & Jensen, 1984; Olds et al., 1984)

Preparing for labor and delivery

The following are appropriate areas for client education to assist the client in reducing her anxiety throughout her last trimester about labor and delivery.

Relaxation exercises are of many types—muscle progression exercises, breathing exercises, visualization exercises, and meditation exercises. Teaching your client any or several of these methods and having her practice them each day prior to labor and delivery will help her use them more effectively during labor. For example, in the muscle progression exercises the client tenses one group of muscles at a time and then relaxes them. The client begins with the feet and progresses *slowly* up the body until all muscle groups have been tensed and relaxed several times. A benefit here is that the client learns an effective method of relaxation and will have taught herself how to let her body totally relax after muscle tensing. The same principles will apply when the client is experiencing intermittent contractions during labor, i.e., muscle tenseness followed by muscle relaxation.

Visual imagery is another simple relaxation technique, done for a few minutes at a time. With visual imagery the client closes her eyes and imagines a pleasant experience from her past or a favorite vacation spot.

In addition, the nurse can encourage the following activities to assist the client in preparation for labor and delivery:

Reading literature designed for expectant parents describing the birthing process.

Participation in expectant parent classes to learn about the birthing process, breathing techniques, and timing contractions. Participation in expectant parent classes can also provide the individual/couple with group support from other couples having a similar experience.

The nurse can also relieve some of the client's concerns by informing the client that:

She may be able to have support systems during labor and delivery, i.e., family and nursing staff. They can provide her with support verbally, nonverbally through the use of touch, etc.

She will receive coaching from the nursing staff as she progresses through each stage of labor.

Medication may be used to assist her in coping with the contractions. Her physician, nurse midwife, or nurse may recommend a medication at a particular time on the basis of how she is progressing and tolerating the process. She should ask the rationale for their recommendations before making her decision.

(Bobak & Jensen, 1984; Olds et al., 1984)

When discussing labor and delivery with clients, avoid using the word "pain." "Pain" creates a negative image for most people. Mrs. Williams perceives the arrival of her child as generally positive, but she has expressed fears about pain. Substituting the terms birthing process and contractions for "pain" may help in reducing her concerns (Olds et al., 1984).

Preparation for breastfeeding

Before discussing preparation for breastfeeding, explore Mrs. Williams's rationale for changing her mind. Help her base her decision on sound data. Support her decision if her rationale is appropriate; e.g., if Mrs. Williams says, "My husband wants me to," she may need some help in exploring the decision further to be sure it is one she will be comfortable with. A discussion of preparation for breastfeeding may not be appropriate at this time if the woman has not raised it as a concern. It would be a priority to follow up with Mrs. Williams within a week to learn her decision. If it is to breastfeed, begin discussion of breast preparation (Bobak & Jensen, 1984; Olds et al., 1984).

Content for teaching	*Rationale*
Supportive brassiere that: • Has wide, nonelastic straps. • Has cups that will support all breast tissue. • Can be enlarged as the chest circumference increases. • Will support the nipple line equidistant between shoulder and elbow without pulling the back of the brassiere up.	To protect breast tissue and prevent sagging. She may be able to use this bra after delivery as well depending upon weight loss.
Encourage her to have the brassiere fitted. (Olds et al., 1984, p. 260)	Many stores have trained personnel who can help clients select a bra that is appropriate for their body build and condition.

Content for teaching	*Rationale*
Skin care: gentle daily cleansing with water; avoid use of soap.	Cleansing will remove hardened colostrum; soap will cause nipples to crack.
Nipple toughening: use friction from bath towel after bathing; nipple rolling between fingers; oral stimulation by partner.	All of these activities will toughen the nipple tissue. However, they should be done in moderation and not to the point of irritation (Olds et al., 1984).
Reading on breastfeeding.	By reading about breastfeeding the expectant mother becomes more knowledgeable about the process and subsequently feels more confident approaching it.

Client education is a major role of the nurse when working with well individuals, families, and groups. To be effective in the teaching role, the nurse needs to have a sound understanding of what facilitates the client's learning and the principles of effective teaching. Pohl (1968) outlines the principles of both learning and teaching as well as their application to nursing as follows:

Principles of learning (Pohl, 1968, pp. 8–26)	*Application to nursing* (Pohl, 1968, pp. 8–26)
1. *Perception is necessary for learning.* The individual needs to be aware of environment.	1. Illness and stress can alter perception.
2. *Conditioning is a way of learning.* Stimuli produce a specific response; habits and attitudes are a response to conditioning.	2. Through positive reinforcement for positive habits/attitudes, the nurse can help the client continue to strengthen them.
3. *The process of trial and error is a way of learning.* We all use this process at times, but it can be wasteful of time and energy.	3. The nurse has a broader knowledge base than the client; helping the client avoid trial-and-error methods can decrease frustration.
4. *Learning may occur through imitation.* Individuals imitate both positive and negative behaviors.	4. The nurse should provide the client with a role model for positive behaviors.
5. *The development of concepts is part of the learning process.* Concept development occurs in the client's mind based on perception, emotions, words, facts, and ideas and results in a meaningful image of some idea, event, place, etc.	5. The nurse can provide the client with information, i.e., pieces of the concept, and answer questions for clarification; however, the integration of perception, emotions, etc., can only occur within the client's mind.
6. *An individual must be motivated to learn.* The individual	6. The nurse may have to help the client identify why he or

Principles of learning
(Pohl, 1968, pp. 8–26)

must want to learn; the desire to learn must be stronger than other drives if learning is to take place.

7. *Physical and mental readiness are necessary for learning.* The physical and mental developmental stages of the client must be considered.

8. *Effective learning requires active participation.* We learn best by doing.

9. *New learning must be based on previous knowledge and experience.* Learning is progressive, always building new ideas on old ones.

10. *The emotional climate affects learning.* Strong emotions, both positive and negative, have an impact on how well we learn.

11. *Repetition strengthens learning.* Using the information helps the individual to learn more effectively and to understand more completely what has been learned.

12. *Satisfaction reinforces learning.* Feeling good about learning can come from within the individual or externally from receiving praise.

Application to nursing
(Pohl, 1968, pp. 8–26)

she is not interested in learning.

7. Illness and/or stress can delay readiness; this should not be confused with lack of motivation.

8. The nurse needs to make the client an integral part of the learning process.

9. The nurse needs to assess each client's knowledge and experience individually and proceed from there. For example, one teaching plan for breastfeeding will not meet the needs of all pregnant clients.

10. The nurse needs to assess the client's emotional status to determine whether teaching is appropriate. The client under extreme stress will not be receptive to learning.

11. The community health nurse can provide reinforcement over time that the hospital nurse cannot.

12. The nurse can provide positive reinforcement by praising the client's progress and can also identify benchmarks for the client as a guide to exactly what and how much has been learned.

Principles of teaching
(Pohl, 1968, pp. 28–45)

1. *Good nurse-learner rapport is important in teaching.* The interpersonal relationship between nurse and client can affect the client's learning.

Application to nursing
(Pohl, 1968, pp. 28–45)

1. Each client should be approached as a unique individual. The client who feels the nurse is genuinely interested in him or her may be more motivated to learn.

Principles of teaching (Pohl, 1968, pp. 8–26)	**Application to nursing** (Pohl, 1968, pp. 8–26)
2. *Teaching requires effective communication.* The learner must understand what the teacher is saying and should feel comfortable about asking for clarification. Miscommunication leads to ineffective teaching; the nurse should avoid using unfamiliar terminology and should be sensitive to the client who has difficulty hearing or for whom English is a second language.	2. The nurse has the opportunity to teach clients how to take care of themselves in terminology they understand and in settings where they feel comfortable. The nurse may need to have clients repeat in their own words what they have perceived.
3. *Learning needs of clients must be determined.* Assessment of learners helps identify their level of present knowledge and what they need to be taught.	3. Through individual assessment the nurse can identify what the client needs to learn, thus avoiding repetition of information the client already knows and understands.
4. *Objectives serve as guides in planning and evaluation of teaching.* These are statements that indicate exactly what the client will be able to do as a result of the nurse's teaching. Objectives are the same as client outcomes.	4. Clear objectives (client outcomes) can be shared with the client, thus allowing the client to know what to expect. Some objectives will be preplanned (as with a group); others will be developed spontaneously as teaching opportunities arise. Preplanning what and how you're going to teach will increase your success in teaching.
5. *Planning time for teaching and learning requires special attention.* Determining when teaching will occur requires forethought and flexibility, both with individuals and with groups.	5. The needs of the client will at times outweigh the nurse's desire or plan to teach.
6. *Control of the environment is an aspect of teaching.* Interference from the environment, i.e., noise, other individuals, poor lighting, etc., can interfere with learning.	6. The nurse can control the teaching environment to a great degree by eliminating noise, distractions, etc.; for example, asking the client to turn off the television during the home visit.
7. *Learning principles must be applied appropriately.* The teacher's success will be	7. The nurse needs to be cognizant of the client's perception, motivation, stress level,

Principles of teaching (Pohl, 1968, pp. 8–26)	**Application to nursing** (Pohl, 1968, pp. 8–26)
directly related to how well the principles of how people learn are used.	readiness and ability to learn. The best-laid plans will fail if the client cannot or refuses to learn.
8. *Teaching skill can be acquired through practice and observation.* Knowing how to teach doesn't "just happen"; it requires motivation, observation, discussion, practice, feedback, and evaluation.	8. The nurse understands that clients learn through trial and error and must feel comfortable doing the same.
9. *Evaluation is an integral part of teaching.* The teacher needs to be able to determine whether he or she has been effective in helping people learn.	9. The nurse can ask, "Did I accomplish what I said I would?" If the objectives (client outcomes) are stated clearly, both the nurse and the client should be able to determine whether the outcomes have been achieved.

As you read through the principles of learning, you will probably be able to identify many that relate to Mrs. Williams and her concerns about the birthing process and breastfeeding; for example:

1. *Perception is necessary for learning.* Mrs. Williams is keenly aware of her pregnancy, her changing body, and her need for information.
2. *Conditioning is a way of learning.* Mrs. Williams has conditioned herself to ask questions and obtain the information she needs.
5. *The development of concepts is part of the learning process.* Mrs. Williams is thinking conceptually when she asks about the pain and how she can help herself. She realizes that her apprehension (fear) regarding the pain will affect her entire body and the labor process. She is asking for new concepts (relaxation) for immediate use and to condition herself for the birthing process.
6. *An individual must be motivated to learn.* Mrs. Williams is motivated. She's asking questions and she's attending expectant parent classes; she wants to learn.
7. *Physical and mental readiness are necessary for learning.* Physically, Mrs. Williams feels and sees her body change as she is in her third trimester. By asking for information on relaxation she's also indicating that she wants to enhance her physical readiness. Her mental readiness is exhibited by her questions; at this point she "expresses concerns." Mild stress can enhance learning; too much stress could prevent her from learning.
8. *Effective learning requires active participation.* Mrs. Williams wants to be involved because she's motivated to learn. She is attending expectant parent classes and is anxious to "help herself."
9. *New learning must be based on previous knowledge and experience.* Mrs. Williams has not had prior experience with pregnancy and has limited information regarding the questions she has asked. Your approach to her with this pregnancy will (may) be different from your

approach in subsequent pregnancies, when you can draw on her experience.

Resolution

Mrs. Williams was responsive to the nurse's suggestion that she learn relaxation techniques. She used the techniques during the remainder of her third trimester and found them to be beneficial in reducing her stress level. She also found they helped her relax during labor.

Mrs. Williams and her husband continued to attend expectant parent classes and found them useful in preparing them for their birthing experience.

Mrs. Williams was admitted to the hospital one week after her due date in true labor and delivered a healthy baby girl. She began breastfeeding without difficulty and is planning to continue breastfeeding until the baby is 5-6 months old.

References

Archer, S. E., & Fleshman, R. P. (1979). *Community health nursing.* (2d ed.) Belmont, CA: Wadsworth.

Bobak, I. M., & Jensen, M. D. (1984). *Essentials of maternity nursing.* St. Louis: Mosby.

Elkins, C. P. (1984). *Community health nursing skills and strategies.* Bowie, MD: Brady.

Hymovich, D. P., & Barnard, M. U. (1979). *Family health care.* (vol. 1) New York: McGraw-Hill.

Olds, S. B., London, M. L., & Ladewig, P. A. (1984). *Maternal-newborn nursing.* (2d ed.) Reading, MA: Addison-Wesley.

Petze, C. F. (1984). Health promotion for the well family. *Nursing Clinics of North America* 19(2):229–237.

Pohl, M. L. (1968). *Teaching function of the nursing practitioner.* Dubuque, IA: Brown.

Shamansky, S. L., & Clausen, C. L. (1980). Levels of prevention: Examination of the concept. *Nursing Outlook* 28(2):104–108.

Stuart, G. W., & Sundeen, S. J. (1983). *Principles and practice of psychiatric nursing.* (2d ed.) St. Louis: Mosby.

Tegtmeier, D., & Elsea, S. (1984). Wellness throughout the maternity cycle. *Nursing Clinics of North America* 19(2):219–227.

SITUATION 10
What Do I Do Now?
(Self-Paced)

SECTION 10.1

You are a staff nurse at the Marion City Department of Health. You have received a referral from a local obstetrician for Barbara Miller, a 23-year-old primigravida in her fourth month of pregnancy. Barbara and her husband, Tom, are high school graduates and live in an apartment. Tom works the night shift full-time on an assembly line in a plastics factory, through which they have insurance coverage. The following problems are listed:

1. Pregnancy – gravida 1, para 0
2. Poor nutritional status
3. Minimal weight gain in pregnancy
4. History of heavy smoking – 2 packs a day

Her physician has made the following comments:

> "Barbara Miller is a new patient whom I have seen once. She has agreed to this referral for home visits by the community health nurse. I would like the community health nurse to do antepartum teaching with emphasis on teaching nutrition, specifically a well-balanced diet. In addition, please work with her to decrease the number of cigarettes smoked. Unfortunately, despite the above problems which I have discussed with Barbara, she does not see herself at risk during this pregnancy."
> Signed: Robert Warner, M.D.

You plan to make a home visit to Barbara this afternoon. She has no phone, so you are unable to notify her of your visit in advance.

You arrive at Barbara's apartment at 2 p.m. Her husband meets you at the door. He says that Barbara is in the living room and asks you to follow him. As you walk through the large kitchen, you notice the environment. The kitchen is furnished with a few cupboards, a sink, an old refrigerator, a small gas stove, and an old wooden table and chairs. The sink is full of dirty dishes. There are also dirty dishes on the kitchen table along with a half-empty bottle of soda, a ham that has been partially eaten, half a loaf of bread, and an open jar of mayonnaise. The ham, mayonnaise, and a greasy frying pan on the stove are covered with flies. The cupboard doors cannot be closed, as the little available cupboard space is filled beyond capacity. The linoleum floor has many stained areas and is sticky beneath your feet. Under the kitchen table is a cardboard box covered with a screen; in the box are two full-grown rabbits.

The living room is a large, drafty room. The windows have shades but are without curtains. Two cats lie sleeping on the window sills. This room is sparsely furnished with several old overstuffed chairs, a sofa, and a television. Barbara is sitting on the sofa in her nightgown, smoking a cigarette and watching a television soap opera. Barbara pushes two more cats off the sofa and offers you a seat. (It's the only available place, as each of the chairs is piled high with blankets and clothes.) There is a heavy odor of cigarette smoke in the air as well as the odor of the animals.

In the work space provided:

a. In your own words describe how you think you would feel in this environment and why.
b. Do you think you can work effectively with Barbara in this environment? State your rationale.

Student Work Space

Turn to the following pages to compare your answers.
a. how you would feel – p. 144
b. work effectively? – p. 145

SECTION 10.2

During your visit with Barbara you gather a comprehensive data base and find out the following related to Barbara's health care problems:

1. **Pregnancy – gravida 1, para 0**

   Subjective data. Barbara states that this pregnancy was not planned but now that she is pregnant she's happy about it. She says she and Tom had been talking about having a baby for several months before she realized that she was pregnant. Barbara says she's looking forward to having a "kid" around; she thinks it will be fun; either a boy or girl will be fine as long as it's healthy. Her husband agrees with each of her comments.

   Objective data. According to referral Barbara is four-and-a-half months pregnant; weight gain is four pounds.

Assessment. Barbara and Tom seem genuinely happy about the pregnancy; they are looking forward to being parents.

2. **Poor nutritional status**
3. **Minimal weight gain**

These two problems will be addressed simultaneously because they are so closely related.

Subjective data. Barbara admits to eating only one balanced meal a day and says she has about eight cups of black coffee throughout the day. She says she does not want to gain a lot of weight with this pregnancy; she says she gains weight easily and has difficulty losing it. In the past, smoking has helped her keep her weight under control. When discussing her dietary intake for today, Barbara indicates she has had the following:

> Breakfast – two cups of black coffee
> Mid-morning – two cups of black coffee
> Lunch – one-half ham sandwich
>   one-half glass of diet soda
>   one cup of black coffee
> Dinner – Barbara says she plans to have scrambled eggs, toast, and black coffee.

When asked about the four food groups, Barbara says she learned about them in school but doesn't pay much attention to them. Barbara says as long as she feels well she is sure the baby will be fine. Husband says he thinks she doesn't eat nearly enough and drinks too much coffee.

Objective data. Barbara is 5'3" and weighs 106 lb; her weight prior to pregnancy was 102 lb. Barbara's color is pale; facial skin is slightly dusky.

Assessment. Barbara has little understanding of what the foods she is eating contain or what constitutes a well-balanced meal; she doesn't seem to understand that her poor nutritional habits will affect her baby; she also is adamant about not wanting to gain weight. Husband seems concerned about Barbara's eating patterns.

4. **History of heavy smoking – 2 packs a day**

Subjective data. Barbara admits to smoking 1½-2 packs of cigarettes a day and says she has no intention of stopping. She says smoking has helped her control her weight since she was 15 years old, and she does not want to gain any more than she has to with this pregnancy. She also says she likes to smoke as it relaxes her.

Barbara admits to a frequent cough but denies any sputum production; she denies dyspnea on exertion. When discussing smoking, she says she knows smoking causes lung cancer but says there is no history of cancer in her family. When asked about the effects smoking can have on her baby, she states that she doesn't think smoking has any effect on the baby. She says that both of her sisters smoked during their pregnancies and their kids are fine. She again admits she wants a healthy baby and reiterates that as long as she feels fine the baby will be fine. Her husband says he has tried to get her to stop; he says she won't believe him when he says it's not good for the baby.

Objective data. Barbara's color is pale, facial skin is slightly dusky. Respirations are 22, even, and not labored.

Assessment. Barbara has a poor understanding of the effects smoking can have on her baby and of the long-term effects smoking can have on her own health; she does not want to stop smoking.

In the work space provided:

a. Identify whether or not you think teaching is appropriate with Barbara. State your rationale.

b. If no, stop here.
   If yes, assess Barbara as a learner by using the principles of learning listed on pages 133–134. State your rationale for each principle selected.

c. With which problem on Barbara's problem list would you begin teaching, and why?

Student Work Space

Turn to the following pages to compare your answers.
a. is teaching appropriate? – p. 146
b. assess Barbara as a learner – p. 148
c. where to begin – p. 149

SECTION 10.3

It is one week later. You arrive at Barbara's apartment. You have prepared a teaching plan you think is specific to Barbara's needs.

As you begin your visit, you sense that Barbara is distracted. You ask her if there is anything bothering her. Barbara tells you that her husband was laid off from his job this morning; he went to the unemployment office a couple of hours ago and hasn't returned. She says she does not think unemployment money will be enough to pay for rent, food, and her doctor's bills.

In the work space provided:

a. State whether or not you think you should continue with your teaching as planned. Support with rationale.

b. In your own words, write what your initial response would be to what Barbara has told you.

c. Are there other community resources (in addition to your own agency) that would be appropriate for Barbara at this time? If yes, list and describe the services.

Student Work Space

Turn to the following pages to compare your answers.
a. continue teaching? – p. 150
b. initial response – p. 151
c. referral – p. 152

SECTION 10.4

It is one week later. You are anxious to see Barbara to find out how she and her husband are managing. In your mind, you review the areas on which you want to follow up and the areas you want to focus on for teaching.

When you arrive at Barbara's apartment there is no response to your knock. You knock several times but there is still no response. As you are writing a note to Barbara to leave on the door, a woman in the next apartment opens her door and says to you, "The people you want to see moved out three days ago." She says none of the neighbors knows where the couple have moved; they left no forwarding address with any of them.

In the work space provided:

a. In your own words describe how you think you would feel in this situation and why.

b. State whether or not you think you have any further obligation to this client. Support with rationale.

Student Work Space

Turn to the following pages to compare your answers.
a. how you would feel – p. 153
b. further obligation – p. 154

ANSWERS TO SECTION 10.1

a. In your own words describe how you think you would feel in this situation and why.

Describing one's feelings in a situation like this is not easy. Some of you may be hesitant to write what you are feeling—hesitant because of what others may think, because you are certain you are alone in your feelings, or because you are embarrassed by your feelings.

Traditionally, nurses are viewed by the general public as helping, caring, feeling professionals. Yet there are times when the feelings experienced by the nurse are not positive, understanding, or empathetic. Instead, feelings of discomfort, frustration, hostility, or even anger may be generated. Nurses are not immune to personal feelings while in a professional role, nor should they be. Feelings are an integral part of each of us as human beings and are often the first indicators which clue us into whether a situation is positive or negative. When feelings of discomfort, frustration, hostility, or anger arise, they should be acknowledged and explained. Our feelings do affect what we say and do and they should not be ignored (Stuart & Sundeen, 1983). At the same time, these feelings should not be the basis upon which decisions regarding clients are made. It is not appropriate for the professional nurse to make judgments regarding clients solely on a feeling level.

If you said you think you would feel uncomfortable, frustrated, or overwhelmed by the environment in which Barbara lives, your feelings are not unusual. Some of you may not feel comfortable in admitting your feelings, but it is only through acknowledging feelings that you can begin to understand them and find effective ways of dealing with them.

Those of you experiencing this type of situation for the first time may question, "Will these feelings disappear?" Yes and no. Feelings of frustration and discomfort are not unusual, particularly when we find ourselves in situations and/or settings that are unfamiliar and/or different from our own life-styles. The majority of nurse-client interactions take place in an environment familiar to the nurse and one in which the nurse has some level of control, i.e., hospitals, nursing homes, physicians' offices, and clinics. Within these settings certain standards will be met, i.e., there will be adequate furnishings and the area will be kept meticulously neat and clean. It is the nurse who sees that the standards are maintained (Lentz & Meyer, 1979).

The home visit, on the other hand, reverses the nurse-client interaction in that it is the client who is in a familiar environment. Whether the environment is clean or dirty, organized or cluttered, the fact remains that it is familiar and comfortable to the client (Barkauskas, 1983). The nurse is a guest of the client, and the client/family maintains control. Initially, the lack of control over the environment can be frustrating to the community health nurse. With exploration of feelings with a peer or supervisor, and with growing maturity and experience, the nurse becomes less concerned with differences in life-style and environment and can focus primarily on the client. This does not mean that the nurse becomes desensitized to differences in life-style and environment. The nurse remains aware but is able to put personal feelings aside and accept the client on his or her own terms.

b. Can you work effectively in this environment?

This question is as challenging as the previous one. It is a question intended to stimulate you to think about how you might feel working with individuals whose values are different from yours. Some of you may think you can work effectively with Barbara within her home environment while others may not. In either case, the rationale you have given can give you some insight into yourself and those things that are important in your value system.

Is there a right answer to the question? Not necessarily. It would be unrealistic to think there could be one right answer to a question that addresses values and value systems. When people find themselves in situations that force them to examine their own value systems and/or attempt to understand the value systems of others, it is not unusual for more questions to be raised than answered. Values are defined by Stuart and Sundeen (1983, p. 66) as "the concepts that a person holds worthy in his own personal life. They are formed as a result of one's life experiences with family, friends, culture, education, work, and relaxation." Value systems are described in the same citation as "more than statements of what one treasures or highly regards. They provide a framework, either consciously or unconsciously, for many of one's daily decisions and actions." Choices and behaviors reflect the unique life experiences of the individual.

A nursing student with limited experience in visiting clients in their homes may wonder, "How will I know if my concern with environment is a conflict in values as opposed to a problem that can be alleviated through my intervention?" Lentz and Meyer (1979, p. 592) suggest the following questions for this analysis:

1. What is the problem with the environment?
2. What has caused this problem?
3. What are the possible remedies?
4. Are these remedies feasible? Can the nurse or the inhabitants realistically implement these changes?
5. What are the less obvious implications in changing the status quo?
6. Who is going to benefit from changing the environment: the client or the nurse?

By taking time to address each of these questions, the nurse can differentiate between an environment that endangers the client's health and one that is simply in conflict with the nurse's values. In the first case, the nurse can (and should) look for ways to change the environment; in the second, attempting change would be inappropriate. If, when thinking about the above questions, it becomes clear that your values are in conflict with the client's in this situation, then other questions may come to mind. For example, "Does a conflict in values mean there is something wrong with my values?" "Does it mean I will be unable to work effectively, as a professional, with this client?"

A conflict in values does not indicate that there is something wrong with the nurse's value system or that the nurse will not be able to work effectively with the client. The conflict signals only that there is a difference in life-style between the nurse and the client. How the conflict is approached by the nurse will determine the nurse's effectiveness with the client. If the conflict is approached in a way that implies that the nurse has negative feelings about the client or is ignoring the client's values altogether, the results are likely to be nonconstructive, generating anger and hostility. Uustal (1978, p. 2058) says that the price paid for not examining one's own values or recognizing conflicts in values often is confusion, indecision, and inconsistency.

On the other hand, the nurse who approaches the client positively will be able to identify effective ways of working with the client within the client's value system (Coletta, 1978). Observed in the home environment, the client becomes a "real person" with interests, hobbies, a culture, family relationships, and values (Keeling, 1978). Seeing the client at home helps the nurse to plan realistic care around those things that are important to the client and his or her family.

For those interested in learning more about values clarification, there are numerous exercises available (Uustal, 1978; Fry, 1985) that can be done alone or in small group discussions. Discussions with faculty and peers can be stimulating and may help to clarify individual thoughts and questions. Understanding one's own personal values and value systems and being comfortable with them enable the nurse to work effectively with clients whose value systems differ.

ANSWERS TO SECTION 10.2

a. Is teaching appropriate with Barbara?

If you answered no, your rationale may be that because Barbara's health-damaging behaviors are an integral part of her daily life, any attempt to teach her would be futile. This rationale prejudges Barbara; it is based primarily on subjective data, possibly on an intuitive level. *It is an inappropriate rationale at this point in the nurse-client relationship.* Please continue reading.

If you answered yes, you are correct. Barbara has three health problems, each of which is a danger to her pregnancy and the child she carries. It is likely that the teaching role with this young woman will not be an easy one, because her nutritional patterns and her smoking are an integral part of her daily life; long-standing behaviors are difficult to change.

Barbara's health-damaging behaviors can be a source of frustration to the nurse who is attempting to do antepartum teaching and to help Barbara with her medical problems. With the frustration comes the question: *Can you change someone else's behavior?* No, you cannot change another person's behavior—that's up to the individual. Families, friends, and health professionals can have a positive influence by confronting the individual with his or her behavior, acquainting him or her with the hazards of continuing the behavior, and modeling an alternative behavior, but the fact remains: the actual change has to come from within the individual.

In this situation with Barbara there *may be* room for change based upon the following reasons:

1. Her pregnancy was planned.
2. She says she wants to have a healthy baby.
3. She does not seem to "have all the facts," i.e., she does not seem to understand how her behavior endangers the health of her baby.

The community health nurse can focus on providing Barbara with the information she is unaware of, specifically the susceptibility of the fetus to Barbara's poor nutritional habits and smoking. On the basis of this new information, perhaps she will then make a more informed decision.

Hochbaum, Kegeles, Leventhal, and Rosenstock (Rosenstock, 1974) have developed a framework called the Health Belief Model, which attempts to explain what motivates people to seek ways to prevent illness—in essence, to change their behavior. The Health Belief Model (Rosenstock, 1974) theorizes that for an individual to seek ways to prevent illness, the individual needs to have three specific perceptions:

1. The individual must *perceive that he or she is susceptible* to a specific disease.
2. The individual must *perceive that contracting the disease would have consequences severe enough to affect his or her life-style.*
3. The individual must *perceive that the benefits* derived from the change in behavior *outweigh the barriers* which have, in the past, prevented this change in behavior.

Variables that may affect these perceptions are the individual's age, culture, sex, and educational background. In addition, the Health Belief Model asserts that the individual can be influenced by *cues to action.* Cues to action may be information obtained from a friend, a health professional, or the media. *Client education can be considered a cue to action.*

Let's apply the components of the Health Belief Model to one of Barbara's medical problems—heavy smoking and its effect on her baby.

1. She *must perceive that heavy smoking puts the pregnancy and/or baby at risk* for specific problems. The pregnancy is susceptible to an increased chance of spontaneous abortion and an increased incidence of placental abruption (Olds, London, & Ladewig, 1984). In addition, there is an increased likelihood that the baby could be stillborn (Bobak & Jensen, 1984), of low birth weight, have a small head circumference, and be shorter in length than the average baby (Da-

vies, Gray, Ellwood, & Abernethy, 1976; Olds et al., 1984). Barbara's statement that she doesn't think smoking has an effect on the baby indicates that she does not understand how susceptible both the pregnancy and the baby are.

2. *She must perceive* that if one (or more) of the above problems occurred in the pregnancy or in the baby, *the consequences would be severe enough to affect her (or the baby's) life-style.* Barbara may learn about the above problems and say, "So what if I have a low-birth-weight baby? He will just be smaller than other babies." A statement like this indicates that she does not understand the implications of having a low-birth-weight baby, i.e., retarded fetal growth (Davies et al., 1976), possible effects on later somatic growth and mental development (Bobak & Jensen, 1984), and possible extended hospitalization in an intensive-care nursery. Other problems sometimes associated with low birth weight are birth defects, blindness, autism, cerebral palsy, and epilepsy (Public Health Service, 1979). With teaching, she may begin to understand the potential consequences and the short-term and long-term effects they could have on her own and the baby's life-style.

3. *She must perceive that the benefits* she will derive from changing her behavior would *outweigh the barriers* which have, in the past, kept her from changing her behavior. In this situation, Barbara is very clear on why she continues to smoke. Her reasons (barriers) are that smoking has helped her control her weight, she likes to smoke, smoking relaxes her, and smoking has been a "habit" for eight years. To overcome these barriers Barbara needs to perceive some significant benefits. Individuals who have successfully stopped smoking have identified the benefits as "feeling better," "looking healthier," and "having greater endurance." It is unlikely that Barbara will see these as benefits. However, what she very well may see as benefits are those directly related to the baby, i.e., delivering a baby of normal birth weight, having a baby whose physical and mental development proceed without delays, or having a baby born alive, not stillborn.

In Barbara's situation, *the cues to action* cannot be emphasized enough. Here the community health nurse has the opportunity to work closely with Barbara and, through client education, help her to see her susceptibility, identify the possible consequences of her smoking, and appreciate the impact they could have on her life-style. In addition, the community health nurse can help Barbara understand the benefits she and the baby would derive if she cut down on her smoking. The community health nurse can then help Barbara confront the barriers that keep her from changing her behavior.

b. Assess Barbara as a learner by using the principles of learning.

The following principles of learning can be readily applied to Barbara as a learner.

Principles of learning (Pohl, 1986)	*Rationale*
Principle 5. The development of concepts is part of the learning process.	Barbara's statement that as long as she feels well, the baby will be fine indicates that Barbara does not understand the total concept of pregnancy, i.e., the dependence of the fetus upon the mother.

Principles of learning (Pohl, 1986)	*Rationale*
Principle 6. An individual must be motivated to learn.	Although Barbara has indicated that she does not want to gain weight, she is happy about the pregnancy and says she wants a healthy baby. Sometimes, the realization that smoking and poor diet actually affect the baby can be a powerful motivator.
Principle 7. Physical and mental readiness are necessary for learning.	Barbara is happy about the pregnancy and looks forward to being a parent. These factors may indicate some level of readiness on her part.
Principle 8. Effective learning requires active participation.	If Barbara is to learn effectively, she needs to be involved in the learning, e.g., deciding what she wants to learn with the nurse. It is then the nurse's responsibility to find creative ways of keeping Barbara actively involved.
Principle 9. New learning must be based upon previous knowledge and experience.	Barbara has had no previous experience with pregnancy except through her sisters. She indicates some level of knowledge regarding the four food groups, but how much is not clear. She shows a minimal level of knowledge regarding the effects of smoking on the fetus.
Principle 10. The emotional climate affects learning.	Both Barbara and her husband are happy about the pregnancy; neither seems to be under major negative stressors. Weight gain and smoking do, however, seem to be emotional issues with Barbara.

c. With which problem on Barbara's problem list would you begin teaching, and why?

The problems on Barbara's problem list are as follows:

1. Pregnancy – gravida 1, para 0
2. Poor nutritional status
3. Minimal weight gain in pregnancy
4. History of heavy smoking—2 packs a day

If you said you would begin teaching with the problem that Barbara would like to work on, you are correct. The most effective learning occurs when the areas identified for teaching are areas in which the client is interested. Teaching imposed by the nurse without regard to the client's interests will result in minimal learning by the client.

Since Barbara has clearly indicated that her eating patterns and her smoking have helped her to avoid gaining weight, it seems unlikely that either of these problems will be problems she chooses to confront. *Some of you may have* used this rationale and *decided to begin teaching with the more general problem of pregnancy*, introducing Barbara to the changes in her body and the growth and development of the fetus. Choosing this strategy could be effective, as Barbara is happy about the pregnancy and does want a healthy baby. The problems of minimal weight gain and smoking can slowly be introduced as part of that teaching. If you have decided to use this approach, your choice is *appropriate.*

Some of you may have decided that the best way to begin teaching with Barbara is to use a direct approach, confronting her with any of the three problems, i.e., minimal weight gain, poor nutrition, or heavy smoking. The process the nurse uses for confronting the client can have a significant impact upon whether the confrontation is effective. For example, an assertive approach may be effective; an assertive approach could contain the following:

1. Some positive reinforcement for Barbara, i.e., it seems she and her husband are happy about the pregnancy, they are looking forward to being parents.
2. Identification of concern by the nurse using an "I" statement, i.e., "I am concerned about these areas."
3. Negotiating with the client to arrive at some compromise, i.e., "Which of these areas would you like to begin with?" or "What do you think would be the best way for me to help you with these areas?"

Although the above approach confronts the issue, it is positive and is likely to elicit some client response. The *assertive* approach acknowledges the individual's feelings and choices and is *appropriate.*

However, if the confrontation is *aggressive* and negative, the client may become angry and disregard the nurse altogether. Clients dislike the nurse who lectures to them about what they are doing wrong (Standeven, 1969). The nurse-client relationship which begins on this tone will be ineffective and the client will not be receptive to learning; this approach is *inappropriate.*

The problems to focus on for client teaching will vary with each situation; one approach is not absolute. The choice is yours!

ANSWERS TO SECTION 10.3 _____

a. Should you continue with your teaching as planned? Support with rationale.

If you answered that you would not continue with your teaching as planned, you are correct. Barbara is *not* ready for teaching—the nurse needs to adapt to this new situation. Once again, the principles of learning and teaching (Pohl, 1968) apply. A quick review of the principles (pages 133–136) as applied to this situation would reveal the following:

Principles of learning (Pohl, 1968)

Principle 1. Perception is necessary for learning. Barbara is distracted by the stressor of her husband's losing his job. She is not completely aware of what is happening around her.

Principle 6. The individual must be motivated to learn. Barbara's present concerns can detract from the interest she showed during the first home visit.

Principle 7. Physical and mental readiness are necessary for learning. Mild stress can act as a motivator for learning. Too much stress can delay readiness. Barbara's distraction by her husband's loss of job indicates that the stressor is significant.

Principle 10. The emotional climate affects learning. Based upon the information Barbara has relayed, it is evident that she has not had sufficient time to adapt to the news of her husband's loss of employment.

Principles of teaching (Pohl, 1968)

Principle 1. Good nurse-learner rapport is important in teaching. The nurse who has a good rapport with the client shows genuine concern for the client's needs. Barbara's needs at this time revolve around her feelings. It would be more appropriate for the nurse to address Barbara's feelings than to attempt any teaching.

Principle 2. Teaching requires effective communication. It is likely that while Barbara is under stress, she will not hear/understand teaching. If Barbara is unable to learn because of the present stressor, the nurse will not be successful in teaching.

Principle 5. Planning time for teaching and learning requires special attention. Timing has to be right for the client; at times, as illustrated in Barbara's situation, the client's immediate needs outweigh the need for teaching.

Principle 7. Learning principles must be applied appropriately. Understanding the learning principles makes the decision regarding whether or not to continue with Barbara's teaching much clearer.

b. Your initial response.

The following would be appropriate as an initial response by the nurse when Barbara talks about her husband's loss of employment and her areas of concern.

> "What a worry for you! Would you like to talk about how you are feeling?"

> "Unexpected changes like losing a job can be very upsetting. Would you like to talk about how you are feeling?"

> "I can understand your concerns. Would you like to talk about them?"

> "I can understand how you feel. Your concerns are very real."

Your initial response to Barbara will be one that facilitates therapeutic communication between you and Barbara. The initial response needs to convey:

1. *Acknowledgment* of Barbara's concerns.
2. *Respect* for Barbara as an individual (Stuart & Sundeen, 1983).
3. *Empathy* regarding Barbara's concerns (Stuart & Sundeen, 1983).
4. *Reassurance* that Barbara's concerns will be addressed.

Acknowledgment of Barbara's concerns conveys to her that the nurse is both listening and hearing what she is saying. Acknowledgment by the nurse needs to be accepting and nonjudgmental in nature. Barbara is likely to continue to express her concerns if she feels the nurse views her concerns as valid. However, if the nurse dismisses Barbara's concerns and feelings as insignificant, Barbara may choose in the future to avoid sharing concerns and feelings with the nurse.

Respect (Stuart & Sundeen, 1983) – valuing the client as an individual. The client's values, culture, beliefs, behaviors, and concerns may differ substantially from those of the nurse, but the concerns Barbara has expressed are valid. The nurse can demonstrate respect for Barbara by acknowledging that her concerns are valid and by showing genuine interest in hearing how Barbara feels.

Empathy (Stuart & Sundeen, 1983) – allowing oneself to feel what the client is feeling. Realistically, the nurse will not always be able to feel what the client is feeling through personal experience. However, the nurse may have had an experience that produced similar feelings. For example, the nurse may never have been laid off from a job but may have terminated one job before securing another, thus producing some similar feelings.

Reassurance that the client's concerns can and will be addressed can be beneficial in reducing stress in the client. Reassurance needs to be sincere and genuine, not patronizing in nature. In this situation, the nurse can reinforce to Barbara the appropriateness of contacting the unemployment service and tell her about additional company resources that can be investigated.

c. Are there other community resources (in addition to your own agency) that would be appropriate for Barbara?

In a situation like Barbara's, where there has been a sudden loss of income, there are additional community resources to which she can be referred. Two specific resources are the Department of Social Welfare and the Women, Infants, and Children Special Supplemental Food Program.

Within the *Department of Social Welfare* each family is assigned a trained social worker. After interviewing the family, the social worker determines whether or not the family or individual members of the family meet criteria for programs administered by the Department of Social Welfare such as the Medicaid program, the Food Stamp program, and/or the Aid to Needy Families with Children program. If the social worker determines family or individual eligibility, then the process of applying for benefits is started.

The Women, Infants, and Children Special Supplemental Food Program (the WIC Program) is a federal program that provides nutritional support to low-income women and children. Established in 1972 as a pilot program, it receives its funding from the Food and Nutrition Service of the U.S. Department of Agriculture (Berkenfield & Schwartz, 1980). In the over ten years of the WIC program's existence, its funding has increased from $20,000,000 a year to over $900,000,000 a year (Rush, 1982). The WIC program is designed to provide supplemental foods and nutrition education to:

- Pregnant women up to six months postpartum
- Nursing mothers up to one year postpartum
- Children from birth to age five (Miller, 1984)

Eligibility of the above groups is based upon income level, geographical area, and nutritional risk. Determining income eligibility is relatively uncomplicated, as guidelines are clearly defined by each state. Geographical location varies, i.e., many states offer services in all geographical areas while others do not. The client needs to live in a geographical area that has been designated to receive funding. Determining nutritional risk is more complex; a nurse or nutritionist interviews the client and reviews the previous medical and nutritional history. Factors which put the pregnant or postpartum woman at risk are:

- Age of the woman, i.e., adolescents or over 40
- Poor obstetrical history such as previous low-birth-weight infants,

miscarriages, short periods between pregnancies, and gestational diabetes
- Anemia
- Poor weight gain (low or high)
- Inadequate consumption of food (Berkenfield & Schwartz, 1980)

Factors which put infants and children at risk are:

- Poor growth
- Anemia
- Obesity
- Chronic illnesses
- Nutrition-related diseases (Berkenfield & Schwartz, 1980)

Based upon the information obtained from the client, the health professional identifies areas of strength and areas for change. A supplemental food package that the client will receive for the next six months is then outlined. The food package will contain foods with high-quality protein, iron, calcium, and vitamins A and C. The specific foods offered tend to be combinations of fruit juice fortified with vitamin C, eggs, milk (low-fat or whole), cheese, fortified cereals, and fortified infant formula (Miller, 1984). Distribution of food packages varies within states. In some states the food is delivered to the home by local dairies; in other states clients receive vouchers that can be exchanged for food packages at local grocery stores.

WIC clients are reevaluated at predetermined intervals. Needs are reassessed, nutrition education continues, and food packages are recertified if appropriate.

ANSWERS TO SECTION 10.4

a. In your own words, describe how you think you would feel in this situation and why.

If you said you think you might feel hurt, disappointed, confused, frustrated, hostile, or angry, you are not unusual. Each of these feelings can be understood. Community health nurses have experienced any combination of these feelings when arriving for a home visit only to find that the client is not at home or, as in this situation, has moved away. Finding clients not at home is less likely to occur with elderly clients who are confined to home with an illness; it occurs more often with young clients. To try to prevent this situation from occurring, the nurse can do several things:

1. Write the date and time of your next visit on a calendar or on a note on the refrigerator in the client's home.
2. If the client has a telephone, call the day before or the morning of the visit as a reminder.
3. Write down your name and phone number so that the client can leave a message for you if the scheduled visit is not convenient or if, as in this case, the family is moving.

When this situation does occur, it is to the nurse's advantage to take time to think about the feelings generated and identify effective ways of resolving them. If feelings are unresolved, they may assume inappropriate proportions, and the nurse may expend large amounts of energy on a situation over which she or he has no control. The nursing student confronted with this situation may benefit from discussing the feelings with the clinical instructor or with other students in a small group.

b. State whether or not you think you have any further obligation to this client. Support with rationale.

This question is likely to generate a significant amount of disagreement. *Some of you may think that the nurse does have a continued obligation to the client and should attempt to find the family.* You are correct. Your rationale may be that the client is high-risk and the relationship has not officially been terminated. Until official termination occurs, attempts definitely need to be made to find the client and continue the relationship.

How much time would be appropriate to spend in attempting to locate her—one phone call? a dozen phone calls? Where would you draw the line? How much time is too much? Is attempting to find the client the best use of your time when you have a responsibility to other clients?

Attempting to locate the client is appropriate. For example, the following actions could be considered:

1. Get in touch with the client's physician by phone or letter explaining the circumstances. Ask the physician to give you the client's address if and when she visits the physician again.
2. Send a written communication to the client at her old address asking her to contact you. Although she did not disclose her new residence to her neighbors, she may have left a forwarding address with the post office.
3. Contact other community resources with which the client may have been involved—for example, the Women, Infants, and Children Supplemental Food Program (WIC) or the Department of Social Welfare. Ask whether they have information they can share with you. However, it is possible that even if these agencies do have information on the client, confidentiality may prohibit the sharing of that information. Should this be the case, it would be appropriate to ask the agency representative to encourage the client to contact you.

What is *inappropriate* is spending inordinate amounts of your time and energy to find the client—time and energy that could be spent more effectively with other clients. When inordinate amounts of time are spent in such activities, the question could be raised, "Who is benefiting from the actions—the client or the nurse?"

Some of you may think that the nurse does not have a continued obligation to the client and that the client record should be closed. Your rationale may include some or all of the following reasons:

1. The client has made no attempt to contact you either by phone, by mail, or by asking her former neighbors to give you her new address. But are you sure of this? Can you be *sure* that the client has not attempted to contact you? No, with the amount of information you have, you cannot be sure that the client has not tried to reach you.
2. The client is responsible for her own actions. Here you are confronting the issue of self-responsibility; the client is an adult and is capable of making personal choices. This rationale is correct. Only the individual can control her choices. Yet, do you know that the client made the move willingly? It is possible that she had little or no warning of the move.
3. Attempting to locate the client may involve too much time. To examine this reason for closing the case, refer to the preceding discussion of time use to determine appropriateness/inappropriateness.

4. The nurse is justified in closing the case because of the frustration and anger it has caused. Although feelings are important and do come into consideration when interacting with clients, those same feelings should not be the basis upon which decisions regarding clients are made. *It is inappropriate for the professional nurse to make decisions regarding clients solely on a feeling level.* If you identified these feelings as your rationale, perhaps taking time to explore those feelings with an instructor or supervisor would be beneficial in clarifying the issue.

What is the right decision in this situation? Some attempts to contact the client can be justified as long as your time and energy permit. If the client is located and chooses to continue the relationship, fine; if she chooses to terminate, you need to respect her choice and allow her to assume responsibility for herself. The referring physician should be notified of your decision and the reason for it.

If the client is not located through the actions previously discussed, then you have no further obligation to the client and the record may be closed. Again, the referring physician should be notified of what occurred.

Resolution

Over a two-week period the community health nurse made numerous attempts to contact Barbara Miller through her obstetrician, the WIC program, and the U.S. mail; all were unsuccessful. None of the agencies/professionals involved with Barbara received any communication from Barbara regarding her change of address or regarding continuing care.

Barbara Miller's record was closed by the community health nurse.

References

Barkauskas, V. (1983). Effectiveness of public health nurse home visits to primiparous mothers and their infants. *American Journal of Public Health* 73(5):573–580.

Berkenfield, J., & Schwartz, J. (1980). Nutrition intervention in the community—the "WIC" program. *New England Journal of Medicine* 302(10):579–581.

Bobak, I. M., & Jensen, M. D. (1984). *Essentials of maternity nursing.* St. Louis: Mosby.

Coletta, S. S. (1978). Values clarification in nursing: Why? *American Journal of Nursing* 78(12):2057.

Davies, D. P., Gray, O. P., Ellwood, P. C., & Abernethy, M. (1976). Cigarette smoking in pregnancy: Associations with maternal weight gain and fetal growth. *Lancet* 1(7955):385–387.

Fry, S. T. (1985). Values and health. In B. W. Spradley (Ed.). *Community health nursing: Concepts and practice.* (2d ed.) Boston: Little, Brown (pp. 106–128).

Keeling, B. L. (1978). Making the most of the first home visit. *Nursing '78* 8(3):24–28.

Lentz, J. R., & Meyer, E. A. (1979). The dirty house. *Nursing Outlook* 27(9):590–593.

Miller, D. F. (1984). *Dimensions of community health.* Dubuque, IA: Brown.

Olds, S. B., London, M. L., & Ladewig, P. A. (1984). *Maternal-newborn nursing.* (2d ed.) Reading, MA: Addison-Wesley.

Pohl, M. L. (1968). *Teaching function of the nursing practitioner.* Dubuque, IA: Brown.

Public Health Service (1979). Healthy people: The surgeon general's report on health promotion and disease prevention (DHEW Publication No. 79-55071). Washington, DC: U.S. Government Printing Office.

Rosenstock, I. M. (1974). Historical origins of the health belief model. In M. Becker (Ed.). *The health belief model and personal health behavior.* Thorofare, NJ: Slack (pp. 1–8).

Rush, D. (1982). Is WIC worthwhile? *American Journal of Public Health* 72(10):1101–1103.

Standeven, M. (1969). What the poor dislike about community health nurses. *Nursing Outlook* 17(9):72–75.

Stuart, G. W., & Sundeen, S. J. (1983). *Principles and practice of psychiatric nursing.* (2d ed.) St. Louis: Mosby.

Uustal, D. (1978). Values clarification in nursing: Application to practice. *American Journal of Nursing* 78(12):2058–2063.

∿∿∿∿∿∿ SITUATION 11 ∿∿∿∿∿
Off to a Good Start
∿∿∿∿∿ (Group Discussion) ∿∿∿∿∿

You are in your office at Stanton County Health Services; it is 4:45 p.m. Monday. The phone rings. It is the continuing care coordinator from the local hospital. She is calling to notify you that one of your clients, Pamela Lewis, a 24-year-old (gravida 2, para 2), delivered a 6 lb 4 oz baby boy at 6 a.m. this morning; both mother and baby are fine. Pamela is taking part in the early discharge program and will be discharged this evening around 6 p.m., i.e., 12 hours post-delivery. You will need to make a postpartum home visit tomorrow.

During antepartum visits you discussed with Pam your agency services for early discharge, and she is aware that you will be home-visiting daily for four days. In addition, Pam has made arrangements for her mother to visit for a ten-day period to help with household chores and to care for Pam's 18-month-old daughter.

SECTION 11.1 ⎯⎯⎯⎯⎯⎯⎯⎯⎯⎯⎯⎯⎯⎯⎯⎯⎯

As you hang up the phone, your thoughts remain on Pam, the new baby, and the home visit you will make tomorrow.

In the work space provided, answer the following:

   a. *Briefly* state what you think your nursing role will be with this well, expanding family.
   b. *Briefly* state why you think women are participating in early postpartum discharge programs.
   c. Identify what time of day you think would be the most ideal for tomorrow's home visit. *Briefly* state your rationale.

Student Work Space ⎯⎯⎯⎯⎯⎯⎯⎯⎯⎯⎯⎯⎯⎯⎯⎯

SECTION 11.2

One of the aspects of your home visits will be postpartum assessment of the mother.

In the work space provided:

    a. List *four* areas you think are the most important in this initial post-partum assessment of Pam.

    b. *Briefly* describe what you would expect to find in your assessment at this point in Pam's postpartum period.

    c. *Briefly* describe the anticipatory guidance (related to your assessment) you think is appropriate.

Student Work Space

Area of assessment	Expected findings	Anticipatory guidance
1.		
2.		
3.		
4.		

SECTION 11.3 _____

An essential part of the postpartum visit is assessment of the newborn baby. The assessment provides a natural opening for the community health nurse to talk with the mother about her baby, and the care he or she needs. A comprehensive assessment includes many areas, eight of which are identified below.

In the work space provided:

For each of the areas identified describe the teaching you think is appropriate for the community health nurse to provide.

Student Work Space _____

Newborn assessment	*Teaching*
1. Color	
2. Temperature	
3. Fontanelles	
4. Eyes	
5. Cord	
6. Urine/Stools	
7. Bathing	
8. Feedings	

SECTION 11.4

As you arrive for your home visit on the third day, Pam greets you at the door. As she speaks she begins to cry. She says she's glad you have arrived because she wants to talk with you privately before her mother returns from grocery shopping. Pam says she is feeling overwhelmed by exhaustion, frustration, and discouragement, in part because the arrangements she made with her mother do not seem to be working out as planned. Pam says there are three major problem areas and describes them as follows:

> "My mother has virtually 'taken over' care of the new baby (with the exception of feedings) and is not helping me with my 18-month-old daughter or meal preparation."

> "I'm very hesitant to talk to my mother because I'm afraid an argument will start. I really don't want to hurt her feelings, but she isn't giving me the help I need."

> "My mother doesn't think I know how to take care of a baby! She says I feed the baby too often—that every four hours is enough. She says that with her babies, if four-hour feedings didn't hold them, she started them on cereal."

In the work space provided, answer the following:

a. What would you say in your *initial response* to Pam? (Write your exact words.)
b. List the steps you would take in attempting to help Pam resolve the above concerns, specifically the first two.
c. Pam's third concern involves a difference of opinion between Pam and her mother regarding the baby's feeding patterns. What do you think you would say to Pam's mother (write your exact words) and why?

Student Work Space

Suggested Reading

American Red Cross (1979). *Advanced first aid and emergency care.* (2d ed.) Garden City, NY: Doubleday.

Archer, S. E., & Fleshman, R. P. (1979). *Community health nursing.* (2d ed.) Belmont, CA: Wadsworth.

Bobak, I. M., & Jensen, M. D. (1984). *Essentials of maternity nursing.* St. Louis: Mosby.

Cronin, M. J., & Stevenson, J. S. (1979). *Workbook on home management of the "well" expanding family.* Burlington: University of Vermont.

Elkins, C. P. (1984). *Community health nursing skills and strategies.* Bowie, MD: Brady.

Hymovich, D. P., & Barnard, M. U. (1979). *Family health care: Volume Two: Developmental and situational crises.* New York: McGraw-Hill.

Jones, D. (1978). Home early after delivery. *American Journal of Nursing* 78(8): 1378–1380.

McCarty, E. (1980). Early postpartum nursing care of mother and infant in the home care setting. *Nursing Clinics of North America* 15(2):361–372.

McKenzie, C. A., Canaday, M. E., & Carroll, E. (1982). Comprehensive care during the postpartum period. *Nursing Clinics of North America* 17(1):23–48.

Olds, S. B., London, M. L., & Ladewig, P. A. (1984). *Maternal-newborn nursing.* (2d ed.) Reading, MA: Addison-Wesley.

Petze, C. F. (1984). Health promotion for the well family. *Nursing Clinics of North America* 19(2):229–237.

Pointer, P., & Lancaster, J. (1984). Assertiveness in community health nursing. In M. Stanhope & J. Lancaster (Eds.). *Community health nursing.* St. Louis: Mosby (pp. 824–842).

Quistad, C. (1984). Getting mothers and newborns off to a good start. *RN* 47(4):39–43.

Regan, K. (1984). Early obstetrical discharge: A program that works. *Canadian Nurse* 80(9):32–35.

Schwalb, R. (1985). Interview. Burlington: University of Vermont.

Spradley, B. W. (1985). *Community health nursing: Concepts and practice.* (2d ed.) Boston: Little, Brown.

Stuart, G. W., & Sundeen, S. J. (1983). *Principles and practice of psychiatric nursing.* (2d ed.) St. Louis: Mosby.

Tegtmeier, D., & Elsea, S. (1984). Wellness throughout the maternity cycle. *Nursing Clinics of North America* 19(2):219–227.

Williams, P., & Bierer, B. (1984). Wash your hands! *Geriatric Nursing* 5(2):103–104.

Wilson, L. (1984). Getting mothers and newborns off to a good start: How to give baby's first physical. *RN* 47(4):44–48.

SITUATION 12
Pregnant Adolescents: An Aggregate (Group Discussion)

SECTION 12.1

You have recently moved from another state and are looking for employment. As you scan the morning paper you see the following advertisement:

Experienced Community Health Nurse

Private, nonprofit agency seeks community health nurse to develop and implement a community outreach program for pregnant adolescents in Madison County. BSN and minimum of two years' community health experience required. Experience working with aggregates and program planning preferred. Contact R. W. Spencer, R.N., M.S., Supervisor, Madison County Health Services, Springfield, 482-9301.

As you think about your work experience, you reflect on the five years since you graduated from your baccalaureate nursing program:

- Two years' experience in a large medical center, where you rotated between labor and delivery and the postpartum unit.
- Three years' experience in a city health department, where you carried a caseload of maternal-child health clients including many adolescents.

Your thoughts return to the advertised position.

In the work space provided, answer the following:

a. What is an aggregate?
b. Describe how you think the role of the nurse in this job will differ from your roles in the two jobs you have held.
c. Based upon the criteria listed in the advertisement, do you think you qualify for the job? Include rationale with your response written below.

163

Student Work Space_____

SECTION 12.2 _____

You arrive for your interview. The supervisor, Ruth Spencer, takes time to tell you of the assessment she has made and how this job has evolved. Madison County is a rural county with a population of 25,000 people, 8,000 of whom reside in the city of Springfield. The adolescent population is approximately 4,500; 2,300 are female.

A major focus of the Madison County Health Services has been maternal-child health care, yet both the staff and the supervisor think their service to the adolescent population has been inconsistent and ineffective. Some of the reasons for the inconsistency are difficulty locating adolescents, not getting involved early enough, difficulty relating to adolescents, and value conflicts between adolescents and staff. She says that the number of adolescents carrying their babies to term has increased from 15 three years ago to 28 last year. She says the individual in charge of vital statistics for the county health services has pointed out that last year's figure was higher than statistics projected for the nation as a whole; i.e., approximately one million adolescents under age 19 (or 10 percent of all teenage girls) become pregnant in any given year and seven of every ten choose to carry their babies to term (Public Health Service, 1979). On the basis of the above information, the supervisor and the staff think it is appropriate to hire a nurse to work full-time with this adolescent population.

The supervisor then turns to you and says:

> "Based on your experience, tell me why you think pregnant adolescents are a high-risk group."

> "Do you have any personal feelings about working with pregnant adolescents? Please answer honestly."

In the work space provided:

Answer both of the above questions including your rationale.

Student Work Space

SECTION 12.3

You are offered the job and you accept. You know that as you approach this new challenge, the framework you will use is the nursing process. The supervisor has presented you with her assessment based on the past three years of agency experience and agency statistics compared with national statistics.

Knowing you need more data to begin planning a program for pregnant adolescents:

a. *Identify additional sources* from which you would gather data.
b. *Briefly describe the type of data* you would be seeking from the sources identified.
c. *Briefly describe the method(s)* you would use to obtain the data you are seeking.

Student Work Space

SECTION 12.4

As you review the data that you have, the following information is significant:

> According to current statistics, the number of adolescent pregnancies in Madison County has doubled in the past three years and is now slightly higher than the national norm; the percentage of low-birth-weight babies born to those adolescents is slightly higher than the percentage born to older mothers (consistent with national statistics) (Bobak & Jensen, 1984).
>
> Representatives of community agencies and area physicians have expressed frustration in working with the pregnant adolescent population for many of the same reasons previously identified by staff nurses. Representatives express support for a program designed for pregnant adolescents.
>
> Representatives of high schools have expressed frustration at the high dropout rate of the pregnant adolescent. In the past three years only 15-20 percent have returned to school. School officials indicate that in areas where comprehensive programs have been developed for pregnant adolescents and teenage parents, the percentage of those returning to school is substantially higher (Public Health Service, 1979). Representatives express support for a program designed for pregnant adolescents.

Adolescents have stated that the following are areas with which they need help:

- Conflict with parents
- Isolation from friends
- Fear of pregnancy, labor, delivery
- Fear of not having enough money
- Conflict with father of the baby
- Frustration over not being in school
- Fear of being a mother

(Jackson, 1985; Mercer, 1979)

The adolescents listed three things they thought would help them:

1. Nonjudgmental, knowledgeable adults to talk to.
2. A chance to talk with other pregnant girls about their pregnancy.
3. A chance to learn more about their pregnancy.

Your assessment confirms that a comprehensive community outreach program for pregnant adolescents is needed in Madison County.

You have scheduled a meeting with your supervisor. In addition to presenting the above data, you will need to do the following:

a. State the outcomes you think are appropriate for a comprehensive outreach program for pregnant adolescents.
b. Briefly outline your plan for developing such a program. Support your plan with rationale.
c. Describe the role you think you will have with the community agencies and the aggregate.

Student Work Space

Suggested Reading

American Public Health Association (1982). The definition and role of public health nursing in the delivery of health care: A statement of the public health nursing section. Washington, DC: The Association.

Aroskar, M. A. (1979). Ethical issues in community health nursing. *Nursing Clinics of North America* 14(1):35–44.

Bobak, I. M., & Jensen, M. D. (1984). *Essentials of maternity nursing.* St. Louis: Mosby.

Daniels, M. B., & Manning, Đ. (1983). A clinic for pregnant teens. *American Journal of Nursing* 83(1):68–71.

Douglass, L. M., & Bevis, E. D. (1983). *Nursing management and leadership in action.* St. Louis: Mosby.

Guttmacher, A. (1976). *11 million teenagers.* New York: Planned Parenthood.

Horn, B. (1983). Cultural beliefs and teenage pregnancy. *Nurse Practitioner* 8(8):38, 39, 74.

Jackson, J. (1985). Interview, nurse midwife. Middlebury, VT: Parent-Child Center of Addison County.

Kandell, N. (1979). The unwed adolescent pregnancy: An accident? *American Journal of Nursing* 79(12):2112–2114.

Lukes, E. (1984). The nursing process and program planning. *Occupational Health Nursing* 32(5):255–256.

McCormick, M. C., Shapiro, S., & Stanfield, B. High-risk mothers: Infant mortality and morbidity in four areas in the United States, 1973–1978. *American Journal of Public Health* 74(1):18–23.

Mercer, R. T. (1979). The pregnant adolescent. In R. T. Mercer (Ed.). *Perspectives on adolescent health care.* Philadelphia: Lippincott (pp. 245–273).

Newman, B. M., & Newman, P. R. (1979). *Development through life: A psychosocial approach.* Homewood, IL: Dorsey Press.

Olds, S. B., London, M. L., & Ladewig, P. A. (1984). *Maternal-newborn nursing.* (2d ed.) Reading, MA: Addison-Wesley.

Public Health Service (1979). Healthy people: The surgeon general's report on health promotion and disease prevention (DHEW Publication No. 79-55071). Washington, DC: U.S. Government Printing Office.

Smith, D. L. (1984). Meeting the psychosocial needs of teenage mothers and fathers. *Nursing Clinics of North America* 19(2): 369–379.

Spradley, B. W. (1985). *Community health nursing: Concepts and practice.* (2d ed.) Boston: Little, Brown.

Stanhope, M., & Lee, G. (1984). Program planning and evaluation in community health. In M. Stanhope & J. Lancaster (Eds.). *Community health nursing.* St. Louis: Mosby (pp. 201–218).

Williams, C. (1977). Community health nursing: What is it? *Nursing Outlook* 25(4):250–254.

Williams, C. (1984). Population-focused practice. In M. Stanhope & J. Lancaster (Eds.). *Community health nursing.* St. Louis: Mosby (pp. 805–815).

PART IV

Occupational Health

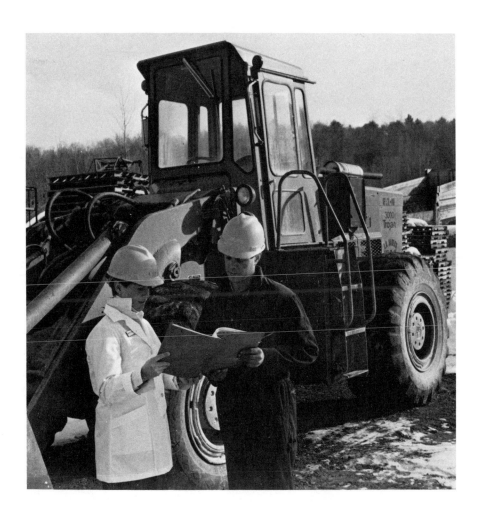

∿∿∿∿∿∿∿ SITUATION 13 ∿∿∿∿∿∿∿
The Employee Physical
∿∿∿∿∿ (Group Discussion) ∿∿∿∿∿

SECTION 13.1 _____

Today, as the occupational health nurse, you have several annual physicals scheduled. The first employee scheduled is John Jones. You review his record before he arrives in your office.

Family Data

		D.O.B.
Employee:	John Jones	9/15/45
Address:	35 Pleasant St., Springfield, U.S.A.	
Spouse:	Mary Jackson Jones	1/5/46
Children:	(1) Cindy *F*	2/3/70
	(2) John *M*	3/1/72

Problem List

1. Health care maintenance
2. Impaired vision *R* eye – legally blind (congenital)
3. Seizure disorder resulting from multitrauma – motor vehicle accident 1963
4. Hypertrophy of gums secondary to Dilantin therapy

Medications

Dilantin 100 mg p/o tid

Hospitalizations

5/8/63 – Multitrauma – motor vehicle accident
12/5/65 – Seizure disorder
5/8/73 – Seizure disorder
8/20/80 – Seizure disorder

Employment Data

Date of employment: 6/5/69   *Department*: Buildings and Grounds
Job description: Involved in general maintenance of the company grounds and maintenance of the interior/exterior of all buildings, i.e., mowing lawns (hand mower); raking leaves; planting/maintenance of shrubbery, lawns, flowers, including spraying of fertilizers and pesticides; painting and light carpentry. All jobs ambulatory in nature.
Activity limitations: May not drive any motorized vehicles, i.e., trucks, cars, forklift, etc. *Exception*: May use a motorized hand-operated lawn mower.

Clinical Findings from Last Year's Physical

B/P – 128/70   Temp 98.4 p/o   Wt 180   Ht 6'1"
P – 70 regular
Respiratory – lungs clear bilaterally   R – 20 even
Abdomen – soft, without masses, active bowel sounds
Peripheral circulation – good, no edema, pulses present
Hearing – within normal limits

Vision – R 20/50 L 20/20   Wears corrective lenses, but vision in R 20/50 even with correction. Peripheral vision R eye absent.
Pupils – R nonreactive L reactive to light
Oral cavity – hypertrophy of gums
Gait and balance – gait steady; good balance
Blood work – CBC within normal limits; urinalysis within normal limits; Dilantin level within therapeutic range.

SECTION 13.2

Clinical Findings from Physical

To be read by faculty member. Use the following space for recording data.

In the work space provided:

   a. State your conclusions about the data you have gathered during this physical.
   b. Is there an area or areas of concern? If yes, identify the area(s). If no, may John return to work?
   c. If you have identified an area of concern, do you need further data to make an assessment? If yes, what type of data do you need and why? If no, state your rationale.

Student Work Space

SECTION 13.3

New Information

To be read by faculty member.

In the work space provided, answer the following questions:

a. Do you agree with Mr. Jones's comments? If yes, state your rationale and stop here. If no, state your rationale and continue.

b. Do you think teaching is appropriate here? If yes, what would you teach? If no, state your rationale.

c. Do you think there is a need for intervention by the nurse? If yes, state your rationale and outline a plan. If no, state your rationale.

Student Work Space

SECTION 13.4

> **New Information**
>
> To be read by faculty member.

In the work space provided:

   a. What are you going to say? (Give an example.)
   b. Does your role end here? State your rationale.
   c. If not, what other action(s) will you take?

Student Work Space

Suggested Reading

Baer, J. (1976). *How to be an assertive (not aggressive) woman in life, in love, and on the job.* New York: Signet.

Brown, M. L. (1981). *Occupational health nursing.* New York: Springer.

Clemen, S. A., Eigsti, D. G., & McGuire, S. L. (1981). *Comprehensive family and community health nursing.* New York: McGraw-Hill.

Hahn, A. B., Barkin, R. L., & Oestreich, S. J. K. (1982). *Pharmacology in nursing.* (15th ed.) St. Louis: Mosby.

Hannigan, L. (1982). Nurse health assessment: The new physical in American industry. *Occupational Health Nursing* 30(8):30–39.

Kinney, M., & Schenk, E. (1983). Problems of the nervous system. In W. J. Phipps, B. C. Long, & N. F. Woods (Eds.). *Medical-surgical nursing.* (2d ed.) St. Louis: Mosby.

Lancaster, J., & Brown, V. (1984). Environmental and occupational health and safety. In M. Stanhope & J. Lancaster (Eds.). *Community health nursing.* St. Louis: Mosby (pp. 285–315).

Malasanos, L., Barkauskas, V., Moss, M., & Stoltenberg-Allen, K. (1985). *Health assessment.* St. Louis: Mosby.

Public Health Service (1979). *Healthy people: The surgeon general's report on health promotion and disease prevention* (DHEW Publication No. 79-55071). Washington, DC: U.S. Government Printing Office.

Speyer, R. (1983). Interview, occupational health nurse, Burlington, VT.

Spradley, B. W. (1985). *Community health nursing: Concepts and practice.* (2d ed.) Boston: Little, Brown.

SITUATION 14
Setting Priorities: Nursing Triage (Self-Paced)

SECTION 14.1

You are the occupational health nurse at XYZ Company, a manufacturer of metal products. You are alone in the office, as your secretary left after lunch to go to a seminar. At approximately 2:30 p.m. five employees arrive at the health office at the same time:

Jack Smith is a healthy 30-year-old man. He works with a piece of machinery that frequently sprays small pieces of metal; safety glasses are required. He is carrying his safety glasses in his hand; they are broken and cannot be worn. He needs new glasses.

Martha Brown is a healthy 25-year-old woman who works in the shipping department; a major part of her job is loading and unloading merchandise from trucks. Martha is ten weeks pregnant. She says she started spotting this morning; the bleeding is starting to increase and she is experiencing a lot of cramping. She says she had a miscarriage one year ago and is afraid she is going to have another one.

Bob Lange is a 56-year-old man with a history of hypertension. He is an executive and under a great deal of stress. He says his physician changed his B/P medication three days ago. Right now he is feeling lightheaded and very dizzy.

John Warren is a supervisor. He is accompanying *Dan Brace*, a healthy 33-year-old man who operates a saw that cuts large sheets of metal; safety glasses are required. Dan is holding a handkerchief against his right eye; there is blood on his face and on the handkerchief; he is in obvious pain. He says there was a malfunction in the saw and a large piece of metal flew up, knocked his glasses off, penetrated his eye, and cut the right side of his face.

In the work space provided:

    a. List the order in which you will see these employees.
    b. State your rationale.
    c. State the directions you will give to the employees you will see second, third, and fourth.
    d. Briefly outline the care you will give to the employee to be seen first. State your rationale.

Student Work Space

Turn to the following pages to compare your answers.
a. order of employees – p. 181
b. rationale – p. 181
c. directions to employees – p. 183
d. care of first employee – p. 183

SECTION 14.2

New Information on Employee Seen Second

Will be found on page 185.

In the work space provided:

    a. State whether or not you agree with the employee's self-evaluation and plan. If yes, state why and stop here. If no, state why and continue.

    b. In your own words, write your response to the employee's plan.

    c. *Briefly* outline a plan for immediate care.

    d. Are there options available for this employee to return to work once stabilized? If yes, what are the options and what is the nurse's responsibility in helping achieve these options? If no, state why.

Student Work Space _____

Turn to the following pages to compare your answers.
a. agree/disagree with employee – p. 185
b. response to employee – p. 186
c. brief plan – p. 186
d. options – p. 188

SECTION 14.3 _____

Employee seen third resolved during care for employee seen second.

> **New Information on Employee Seen Fourth**
>
> Will be found on page 189.

In the work space provided:

a. State whether or not you feel this is an appropriate time for teaching. If yes, briefly outline areas for teaching and your rationale. If no, state your rationale.

b. Can this employee return to work? If yes, state your rationale. If no, state your rationale.

Student Work Space

Turn to the following pages to compare your answers.
a. is teaching appropriate? – p. 189
b. return to work? – p. 191

SECTION 14.4

> **New Information on Employee Seen First**
>
> Will be found on page 191.

In the work space provided:

    a. State how you would respond to this phone call.
    b. State whether or not the nurse's responsibility ends here. State your rationale.

Student Work Space

Turn to the following pages to compare your answers.
a. response to phone call – p. 192
b. nurse's responsibility – p. 192

ANSWERS TO SECTION 14.1

a. List the order in which you will see these employees.
b. State your rationale.

a. Suggested order	*b. Rationale*
1. Dan Brace	1. Penetrating eye injuries are serious and may result in loss of vision or complete blindness. This type of injury should be treated promptly by an ophthalmologist. The sooner the individual receives treatment, the greater the chances are of saving the eye and/or sight (American Red Cross, 1979; Chenoweth & Broseman, 1983).
2. Martha Brown	2. Vaginal bleeding and cramping are signs of possible miscarriage. She indicates the bleeding is starting to increase in volume; excessive bleeding can result in weakness, fainting, and even shock. She can begin providing some of her own care initially while you are providing emergency treatment for Dan's eye injury (American Red Cross, 1979).

You may have put Martha Brown first and Dan Brace second, reasoning that any abnormal bleeding needs to be treated immediately. This rationale is accurate. Martha's care can be started immediately based on your instructions (see answers section 14.1c) so that you can give full attention to Dan's eye injury. Keep in mind that you will provide minimal care for Dan; he needs emergency care from an ophthalmologist, and little time will elapse before you are able to give Martha your full attention.

a. Suggested order	*b. Rationale*
3. Jack Smith	3. This employee has no need for medical treatment but has to return to the production line as quickly as possible. His needs are simple and can be taken care of quickly. Occupational health nurses are aware that in industry increased production and increased profits are the priorities (Silberstein, 1981). Therefore, time away from production is kept to a minimum. However, production and profits *do not* take precedence over the health and welfare of the employee. The needs of Dan Brace and Martha Brown must be attended to first. Jack Smith can be seen before Bob Lange, the man with hypertension, as Bob's situation is not as acute as that of the others but may require a significant amount of the nurse's time. Jack Smith should not return to the production line without safety glasses, as this would compromise his safety and be in conflict with company regulations. In some companies the responsibility for dispensing safety glasses is given to other personnel, such as a safety officer, thus allowing the nurse to use time more efficiently with employees having other needs.
4. Bob Lange	4. This man can be seen last (see above discussion on Jack Smith) provided he is given directions that will begin his care while he is waiting. His need for care is otherwise not as acute as that of Martha and Dan. He may require some teaching, however, which will increase the amount of time the nurse will need to spend with him (American Red Cross, 1979).

In ordering the employees you may have reversed the order of Jack Smith and Bob Lange based on the rationale that Bob Lange has a potentially more serious problem. Although that may be true, he can be given directions that will start his care while the nurse is providing direct care to the others.

In many companies there is a larger nursing staff available than in this situation, and often there is a physician on site as well. In such settings the above employees would have been cared for simultaneously.

c. State the directions you will give to the employees you will see second, third, and fourth.

2. Martha Brown   Direct Martha to an examining room close to a bathroom.
Instruct her to lie down on the bed/stretcher to decrease chances of fainting if bleeding continues. Tell her to elevate her feet.
Tell her where the sanitary pads are located in the examining room.
Tell her that any large clots or tissue passed should be saved.
Let her know you will be with her as soon as possible.

By taking the above actions, the nurse has initiated appropriate care for Martha (Bobak & Jensen, 1984; Olds, London, & Ladewig, 1984).

3. Jack Smith   Tell Jack that he will have to wait until those with acute problems are seen and that you are aware he cannot return to his job without his safety glasses.
Ask him to sit in the waiting area.

4. Bob Lange   Direct Bob to an examining room.
Tell him to lie down to decrease chances of fainting.

d. Briefly outline the care you will give to the employee to be seen first. State your rationale.

Dan Brace – As stated earlier, a penetrating eye injury needs prompt care.

The *assessment* phase of care will be limited. If the eye has been punctured, the nurse *should not* attempt to determine the extent of the injury. The employee needs to be referred for medical care immediately (American Red Cross, 1979).

The following care is suggested:

Talk to Dan while you are providing the following care and let him know what you want him to do as well as what you will be doing for him. In an emergency situation like this the employee can be extremely frightened and/or apprehensive. His stress level can be reduced by providing him with accurate information and efficient care (American Red Cross, 1979).

Care	*Rationale*
1. Keep Dan quiet. It is preferable to have him lie down. At the very least have him sit (American Red Cross, 1979).	1. Preventing unnecessary movement reduces the chance of extending the injury. Movement (walking, bending) will increase intraocular pressure and cause further damage (Chenoweth & Broseman, 1983).
2. Make *no* attempt to remove the object or to wash the eye (American Red Cross, 1979).	2. Either of these actions would increase the damage to the eye (Chenoweth & Broseman, 1983).

Care	*Rationale*
3. Do not cleanse or wipe area surrounding the eye (American Red Cross, 1979).	3. Wiping/cleansing can change intraocular pressure and cause further damage (Chenoweth & Broseman, 1983).
4. Cover both eyes *loosely* with a sterile dressing. Hold dressings secure by using a bandage (Kerlix, Kling) that encircles the employee's head. Avoid any pressure on the affected eye. (To prevent pressure, a metal eye patch or a structure like a paper cup may be used to cover the eye.) (American Red Cross, 1979; Chenoweth & Broseman, 1983)	4. Covering both eyes will decrease movement in the affected eye to a minimum. Pressure on the affected eye will increase intraocular pressure (American Red Cross, 1979; Chenoweth & Broseman, 1983).
5. Notify the nearest emergency room and/or eye specialist that the employee is being transported for emergency care. (Some companies have an ophthalmologist as a consultant who sees all work-related eye injuries.)	5. Prior notification will assure prompt attention/medical care (American Red Cross, 1979; Brown, 1981).
6. Transport the employee to nearest emergency room either by rescue squad or by car. If going by car, transport to car in a wheelchair (American Red Cross, 1979).	6. Arrange immediate transportation for prompt treatment. Transportation by rescue squad may be stress-producing; employee may prefer to be transported by car. Presence of supervisor provides moral support. Keep movement at a minimum to prevent increasing intraocular pressure (American Red Cross, 1979; Chenoweth & Broseman, 1983).
7. Contact family. The nurse can delegate this responsibility to the supervisor while the employee is being prepared for transportation to the emergency room.	7. A family member or significant other can provide support to the injured employee. It is important for the company representative to describe the problem without frightening or angering the family member.
8. Document. The nurse will need to complete an accident report on a form designed for that purpose.	8. See page 192.

Short-term resolution

Dan Brace was transported to the nearby medical center (within ten minutes of entering the occupational health office) by his supervisor. He was met there by his wife and an ophthalmologist. He underwent a lengthy surgical procedure in which the lens of the eye had to be removed; his eye was left with a Y-shaped scar. Subsequently, his vision in that eye was severely limited, i.e., he was only able to distinguish light from dark. Dan remained out of work for a period of two months.

Long-term resolution

Since XYZ Company has a policy of reassigning employees whose capabilities are changed by illness or injury, Dan's job was changed upon his return to work because of his limited vision. At present Dan wears a contact lens in his affected eye but still has minimal vision.

New Information

As Dan Brace leaves the health office with his supervisor en route to the medical center, your thoughts turn immediately to Martha Brown, the next employee to be seen.

Your assessment of Martha reveals the following:

Martha says she feels better than when she came into the health office. She denies weakness or lightheadedness. She says she is experiencing some abdominal cramping but says, "They aren't too bad—they feel like menstrual cramps."

Her B/P is 100/70 (normally 105/76); pulse is 86 and regular (normally 72); respirations are 20 and even (normally the same). Her color is good; her skin is cool and dry. She is alert and oriented. She has two fresh pads in place with approximately 60 cc of bright red drainage. She has saturated three other pads since 10 a.m. that morning.

She says the bleeding is slowing, that she feels "okay," and that she thinks she'll return to work. She says her husband was laid off two weeks ago and she cannot afford to miss any work.

Using the above information, turn to page 178 and answer the questions pertaining to Martha's care.

ANSWERS TO SECTION 14.2 _____

a. Agree/disagree with Martha's self-evaluation and plan.

If you disagree with Martha's self-evaluation and plan, congratulations!

Based upon the data that Martha gives you, there should be no question that her self-evaluation and her plan are inappropriate. Martha needs to be evaluated by her obstetrician.

Reasons	*Rationale*
1. The bleeding has continued and actually increased.	1. Loss of blood can result in hypovolemia and hypovolemic shock.

Reasons	*Rationale*
2. The abdominal cramping has continued.	2. Cramping is indicative of continued uterine contractions not found in the normal pregnancy (Bobak & Jensen, 1984; Olds et al., 1984).
3. There are changes in her vital signs, i.e., B/P and pulse.	3. A decrease in B/P occurs with the loss of circulating volume; an increased pulse occurs as an attempt to increase cardiac output to maintain B/P within normal range. Increased pulse could be related to increased stress, but B/P should remain unchanged or possibly increase (Olds et al., 1984; Cassmeyer, 1983).
4. She has a history of a miscarriage a year ago.	4. With her history and current symptoms she is at risk for a spontaneous abortion.
5. She expresses concern about losing work because her husband was laid off.	5. Her concern is understandable, but returning to work at this time could increase the risk of spontaneous abortion.

If you agree with Martha, reread the situation, then review the data and the above rationale again. It would be inappropriate to allow this employee to return to work (even if she were stable). Brown (1981, p. 4) states that "the primary goal of occupational health nursing practice is to assist the worker to attain and maintain optimal physical and psychological functioning." The work Martha does, i.e., heavy lifting, could continue to affect her well-being and her ability to carry her child to term *even after* she has stabilized. It would be inappropriate to allow an employee to return to work when her health and wellness would clearly be at risk.

b. Response to Martha's plan.

The nurse needs to be firm and assertive in this situation, presenting the assessment and the rationale on which it is based. Martha's concern about her husband's loss of work should be acknowledged as a preface to the response in which the nurse states why Martha should not return to work.

Use of "I" statements will be beneficial here (turn to page 17 for rationale supporting the use of "I" statements). Reviewing with Martha her past history, and current symptoms, the nurse should strongly recommend medical evaluation by Martha's obstetrician (Baer, 1976; Pointer & Lancaster, 1984).

Possible acknowledgments of Martha's concern:

> "I can understand your reason for wanting to return to work."
>
> "I can understand your worries about money."

Referral to an employee assistance program or the Department of Social Welfare for help with financial planning are appropriate to discuss with Martha at this time.

Possible responses regarding Martha's care:

> "I think it would be unwise to return to work for both you and your baby. I want your physician to see you. I will need a written decision from him or her before you return to work."

> "I think it would be in the best interest of both you and the baby if . . ."

> "I cannot let you return to work because my assessment indicates . . ."

> "I want your physician to examine you. I will need a written decision by him or her before you can return to work."

c. Brief plan of immediate care for Martha Brown.

The following is a *suggested* plan of care.

Care	*Rationale*
1. Monitor vital signs, i.e., B/P, pulse, and respirations.	1. Loss of blood can result in hypovolemia and hypovolemic shock. A decrease in B/P occurs with a loss of circulating volume; an increased pulse occurs as an attempt by the body to increase cardiac output to maintain B/P within the normal range. Respirations will increase with decreased circulating volume in an attempt to compensate for the decreased oxygen available (Olds et al., 1984; Cassmeyer, 1983).
2. Monitor color and general strength.	2. Color becomes pale, and client becomes weakened with loss of circulating volume. The body shunts the blood away from the periphery and directs it to the vital organs in an attempt to maintain B/P (Olds et al., 1984; Cassmeyer, 1983).
3. Talk with the employee.	3. Provide her with clear, concise information and tell her what you think the plan of care should be. Encourage her to verbalize her feelings (Bobak & Jensen, 1984; Cassmeyer, 1983).
4. Maintain employee in a reclining position.	4. Feet may be elevated to decrease peripheral resistance of circulating volume; this will also facilitate circulation to the brain (Olds et al., 1984; Cassmeyer, 1983).
5. Monitor loss of blood, i.e., pad count, color of drainage, consistency, etc. (Olds et al., 1984).	5. Loss of blood can result in decreased circulating volume and therefore in decreased circulating oxygen (Olds et al., 1984; Cassmeyer, 1983).

Care	*Rationale*
6. Monitor abdominal cramps, i.e., presence/absence, frequency, intensity, duration.	6. Cramping is indicative of continued uterine contractions not found in the normal pregnancy (Bobak & Jensen, 1984; Olds et al., 1984).
7. Have oxygen therapy available.	7. Loss of blood can result in decreased circulating volume and therefore in decreased circulating oxygen, with possibility of dyspnea, restlessness, or disorientation (Olds et al., 1984; Cassmeyer, 1983).
8. Contact employee's physician.	8. Relay all subjective and objective data that you have. Make arrangements for employee to be seen by physician. (If the employee does not have a physician, the nurse may need to refer her to one. The company may have an agreement with a local obstetrician who will cover such emergencies and who will accept referrals from the occupational health nurse or physician.) (Brown, 1981)
9. Contact family member.	9. Husband, significant other, or family member indicated by employee needs to be informed of the situation.
10. Make arrangements for transporting employee.	10. The employee will need to be transported to the physician's office for examination (or to the emergency room if severe shock is occurring) (Brown, 1981). If the employee can be transported by car, it would be preferable to have a family member provide that transportation as it will be less stressful for the employee. A family member will be able to remain with the employee in the physician's office and will be able to take the employee home. The continuity provided by a family member will help decrease stress for the employee. If a family member is not available, the nurse will need to make arrangements for someone from the company to provide that service. (If bleeding is severe, transportation by ambulance may be necessary.)

d. Options for Martha Brown's returning to work.

There are options that will enable this woman to return to work once she has stabilized and received approval from her physician. She cannot go back to her current job; heavy lifting will only continue to endanger her pregnancy. If she cannot be accommodated in her own department with an activity restriction, she may be given a job in another department.

The nurse has a responsibility to investigate the job reassignment options available to the employee. The nurse may not be able to tell the employee immediately what arrangements can be made but will be able to do so after conferring with the employee's physician and supervisor. The nurse will contact the supervisor and outline the situation, identifying the reasons why modifications need to be made in the employee's tasks (Brown, 1981).

The nurse is responsible for notifying the supervisor and the personnel office in writing of the limitations on the employee's activity. (Each company has specific forms identified for this purpose.) Written validation also needs to appear in the employee's medical record (Brown, 1981).

Resolution

Martha says she knows you are right and that she should not return to work. She agrees to see her physician. You contact Martha's husband and he agrees to transport her to the physician's office.

While waiting for his arrival, you leave Martha resting in the examining room. You fit Jack Smith for a new pair of safety glasses and he returns to work.

Martha was taken to the car in a wheelchair by her husband. She was seen by her physician and spent several days on bed rest before returning to work. Upon her return she was assigned a sedentary job in another department. As a result, she was able to work until two weeks before delivery. She delivered a healthy baby girl.

ANSWERS TO SECTION 14.3 ―――――――――――

New Information

After Martha leaves the health office you enter the examining room where Bob Lange is. You find he is asleep. You check his pulse. It is 76 and regular (normally 72). His respirations are 20 and even. As you place the B/P cuff on his arm Bob wakes up; his B/P is 110/80 (normally 140/88 on Lasix therapy). Bob says he feels much better. He says that ever since his doctor changed his B/P medication from Lasix to Hydralazine he's had episodes of lightheadedness but doesn't understand why. Using the above information, turn to page 179 and answer the questions as they pertain to Bob.

---

a. Is this an appropriate time for teaching?

This is indeed an appropriate time for teaching. A brief review of the principles of learning on pages 133–134 (Pohl, 1968, pp. 8–26) indicates that some of the principles apply to Bob Lange. For example:

Principle 6: *An individual must be motivated to learn.* Bob Lange voices concern about his episodes of lightheadedness and says he doesn't understand what is causing them.

Principle 7: *Physical and mental readiness are necessary for learning.* When physical symptoms are present and the individual's stress level is elevated, learning cannot take place; when symptoms subside and stress level is decreased, learning can take place.

Principle 10: *The emotional climate affects learning.* Bob is relaxed and says he feels much better; his stress level is reduced. He can be more receptive to learning.

In reviewing the principles of learning, are there others you think apply to Bob Lange?

The following are *suggested* areas for teaching, with supporting rationale.

Areas for teaching	*Rationale*
1. Explain the different physiological actions of Lasix (thiazide) and Hydralazine (vasodilator) in simple terms so that he can understand the reason for his lightheadedness.	1. Lasix blocks sodium reabsorption in cortical portion of the ascending tubule; water is excreted with sodium, producing decreased blood volume. Lightheadedness can result if client becomes hypovolemic. Hydralazine relaxes arteriolar smooth muscle causing vasodilation. Vasodilation in the periphery will take some volume from the brain, thus decreasing the supply of oxygen to brain tissue and causing lightheadedness. His body may need several days to adapt to the vasodilation stimulated by the new medication (Hahn, Barkin, & Oestreich, 1982; Daly, 1983).
2. Discuss his medication and how to take it.	2. To increase therapeutic effect.
3. Acquaint him with the possible side effects of his medication, i.e., dizziness, tachycardia, nausea, weakness, angina, rash, fever, headache (Hahn et al., 1982; Daly, 1983).	3. Client should be aware of side effects so that he can report to his physician if any should occur.
4. Tell him to notify physician when side effects occur.	4. To allow physician opportunity to reevaluate.
5. Advise him to have regular checkups with his physician and regular B/P checks.	5. Clients who have hypertension will need medical supervision for the rest of their lives. B/P checks help the client know if he is well regulated or if he needs to be seen by his physician.
6. Suggest that he avoid sudden position changes such as sitting to standing or lying down to standing.	6. Same as #1 – vasodilation.

SITUATION 14 *Setting Priorities: Nursing Triage*   **191**

Areas for teaching	*Rationale*
7. Instruct him not to discontinue B/P medication without a physician's approval.	7. Sudden cessation of B/P medication can result in a hypertensive crisis (Hahn et al., 1982; Daly, 1983).
8. Recommend modifications in diet, i.e., decrease sodium intake, decrease fat intake.	8. Sodium is believed to be a factor in increasing circulating volume and, therefore, increasing B/P. Fats are believed to be a factor in arteriosclerosis, which decreases the lumen of the artery and, therefore, increases B/P (Daly, 1983).
9. Encourage some form of stress management, i.e., meditation, visualization.	9. Stress-producing situations have been related to hypertension. It is believed in some individuals that the general adaptation syndrome may be ineffective and that stress may be physiologically harmful.

b. Can Bob Lange return to work?

Yes, Bob can return to work as long as his symptoms have abated. Since Bob has a sedentary desk job, his return to work would not be hazardous to his safety (in the workplace) should the symptoms recur. Bob should be encouraged to return to the health office if he does not feel well.

If symptoms persist, he should be encouraged to see his physician, as the recent adjustment in his medication regimen may need to be reevaluated.

Many companies have well-established hypertension screening and follow-up programs for their employees. If such a program does exist, he should be encouraged (offered the option) to participate.

Resolution

Bob Lange was receptive to teaching and asked many excellent questions about his medication and its physiological effects. He returned to the health office at the conclusion of the workday and twice the following day to have his blood pressure monitored. (Bob notified his physician of his symptoms.) He adapted to his new medication and the symptoms were alleviated. Bob began regular follow-up in the company hypertension program.

ANSWERS TO SECTION 14.4 ⎯⎯⎯⎯⎯⎯⎯⎯⎯

New Information

After Bob Lange leaves your office, the phone rings. It is Jean Brace, Dan's wife. She says Dan was seen immediately in the emergency room and is now in surgery. She says they have been under a lot of financial strain lately, and she wants to know if his insurance will cover his surgery and if he will receive any sick pay while he is out of work. Turn to page 180 and answer the questions as they pertain to the above conversation with Dan Brace's wife.

a. How would you respond to this phone call?

The nurse can reassure Dan Brace's wife that her husband's surgery and hospitalization will be paid for through workers' compensation insurance. In addition, workers' compensation will also provide him with salary during the time he is unable to work.

The first state workers' compensation legislation was enacted in 1911; by 1948 all states provided such insurance. The primary purpose of the insurance is protection of the employee and the employer. The employer bears the cost of the insurance and maintains a safe work environment for the employee (Brown, 1981).

If a work-related illness/injury occurs, the insurance provides the employee with compensation for medical costs and salary while the employee is unable to work. (Salary compensation may be less than the employee's actual salary.) Additional compensation may be given to the employee based upon the type of injury/illness, its degree, permanence, and the number of dependents the employee has (Brown, 1981; Clemen, Eigsti, & McGuire, 1981).

b. Does the nurse's responsibility end here?

The nurse's responsibility in this situation with Dan Brace does not end here. The following are areas the nurse would need to address:

1. *Accident report.* An accident report is essential (Brown, 1981) to provide the company and workers' compensation with accurate, complete, concise information about the employee's accident. The following areas/questions should be addressed when preparing an accident report:

   - Name, age, and address of the employee
   - Date, time, and location of the accident
   - Description of the accident
   - Names of individuals who witnessed/described the accident
   - Description of the injury sustained
   - Description of the care given to the employee
   - Disposition of the employee, i.e., to home, hospital, with whom, means of transport used
   - Name of the employee who delivered the care/prepared the accident report
   - Name of spouse, relative(s) contacted; date and time of contact

   A similar accident report also needs to be submitted by the employee's supervisor. The reports will become a permanent part of the employee's record, his personnel file, and his file at the workers' compensation office.

   In some companies the nurse is a member of the safety committee (or is the safety officer) and would review the accident in terms of how and why it occurred. For example, was it a freak accident? Was it due to employee negligence? Was it due to defective equipment? Based upon the review, recommendations would then be made to prevent similar occurrences (Brown, 1981).

2. *Benefits.* Because the employee will be away from work for an extended period, he will need to rely on his benefits. It is the nurse's

responsibility to begin the process enabling the employee to receive those benefits. For example: There is generally a time frame in which claims need to be made for coverage by workers' compensation, i.e., 48 hours from the time of the injury. Should problems arise in securing benefits, the nurse may need to serve as an advocate for the employee. Monetary benefits received by the employee from workers' compensation will be less than his previous salary. The nurse may need to act as a resource person in helping the employee determine whether he and his family are eligible for benefits from other community resources (Clemen et al., 1981).

3. *Follow-up.* The nurse will be involved in follow-up over an extended period of time with an employee who has had an injury/illness. The nurse will be concerned with some of the following areas (Brown, 1981; Clemen et al., 1981):

- The employee's ability to return to work in the same or a different job
- Periodic screening to determine loss of function (in this situation, screening of both the affected and the nonaffected eye)
- Teaching on health care maintenance and eye protection

Follow-up by the nurse is an excellent way for the employee and his family to appreciate that the company is concerned with the health of its individual employees.

Resolution

Dan's expenses for hospitalization and surgery were covered by workers' compensation. He received salary compensation during his convalescence. Based upon the degree of Dan's injury and his permanent loss of vision, the state workers' compensation board voted Dan a one-time financial award and agreed to assume responsibility for future medical expenses related to the eye injury.

References

American Red Cross (1979). *Advanced first aid and emergency care.* (2d ed.) Garden City, NY: Doubleday.

Baer, J. (1976). *How to be an assertive (not aggressive) woman in life, in love and on the job.* New York: Signet.

Bobak, I. M., & Jensen, M. D. (1984). *Essentials of maternity nursing.* St. Louis: Mosby.

Brown, M. L. (1981). *Occupational health nursing.* New York: Springer.

Cassmeyer, V. L. (1983). Mechanisms for maintaining dynamic equilibrium. In W. J. Phipps, B. C. Long, & N. F. Woods (Eds.). *Medical-surgical nursing.* (2d ed.) St. Louis: Mosby (pp. 296–325).

Chenoweth, L., & Broseman, L. A. (1983). Problems of special senses: Eye and ear. In W. J. Phipps, B. C. Long, & N. F. Woods (Eds.). *Medical-surgical nursing.* (2d ed.) St. Louis: Mosby (pp. 895–913).

Clemen, S. A., Eigsti, D. G., & McGuire, S. L. (1981). *Comprehensive family and community health nursing.* New York: McGraw-Hill.

Daly, B. J. (1983). Problems of peripheral circulation. In W. J. Phipps, B. C. Long, & N. F. Woods (Eds.). *Medical-surgical nursing.* (2d ed.) St. Louis: Mosby (pp. 1142–1185).

Hahn, A. B., Barkin, R. L., & Oestreich, S. J. K. (1982). *Pharmacology in nursing.* (15th ed.) St. Louis: Mosby.

Olds, S. B., London, M. L., & Ladewig, P. A. (1984). *Maternal-newborn nursing.* (2d ed.) Reading, MA: Addison-Wesley.

Pohl, M. L. (1968). *Teaching function of the nurse practitioner.* Dubuque, IA: Brown.

Pointer, P., & Lancaster, J. (1984). Assertiveness in community health nursing. In M. Stanhope & J. Lancaster (Eds.). *Community health nursing.* St. Louis: Mosby (pp. 824–842).

Silberstein, C. A. (1981). Nursing role in occupational health. In L. L. Jarvis (Ed.). *Community health nursing: Keeping the public healthy.* Philadelphia: Davis (pp. 123–140).

SITUATION 15
A Problem Bigger Than It Seems
(Self-Paced)

SECTION 15.1

You have been the occupational health nurse at Cromwell Computer Company, Inc., for two months. The company has been in operation for approximately fifteen years and employs 600 people. Since the company physician with whom you work is on site just one day a week, you are the primary health care provider.

It is Monday afternoon. The phone rings with a call from one of the floor supervisors. He would like to come to your office to discuss his concerns regarding one of the employees. You agree to meet with him.

The supervisor arrives in your office. He says he is concerned about Ralph Johnson, age 43, an employee who has worked for the company since it opened. The supervisor says he began to notice subtle changes in Ralph's behavior about two months ago: he seemed to forget things easily and began to argue frequently with other employees. In the past month these actions have increased in frequency, and his attendance at work has been inconsistent. The supervisor shows you his documentation of Ralph's recent attendance:

> March 8 – Friday – late 30 minutes
> March 18 – Monday – absent
> April 1 – Monday – absent
> April 4 – Thursday – left work at 11 a.m.; not feeling well
> April 9 – Tuesday – late 15 minutes
> April 11 – Thursday – late 20 minutes
> April 15 – Monday – left work at noon; not feeling well
> April 19 – Friday – late 1½ hours
> (today) April 22 – Monday – late 25 minutes

His prior record of attendance had been very good except for occasional absences (1–2 days a year) due to colds. He had always been noted for his promptness in arriving for work.

The supervisor says he has tried to help Ralph in a number of ways, i.e., making excuses for him, helping him meet his quotas, etc., but Ralph has not been receptive.

The supervisor tells you that he met Ralph in the hall today returning from lunch and for the fourth time in three weeks smelled alcohol on his breath. The supervisor asks you for your help with this situation, as he does not know what to do about it. You refer to the company's policies and find that the policies addressing the employee with a drinking problem are vague and provide you with little direction.

In the work space provided answer the following:

a. Do you think this situation is of high priority? Support your conclusion with rationale. If your answer is no, stop here.

b. If your answer is yes, identify what you think are appropriate actions for the nurse. Support the actions you have selected with rationale.

Student Work Space

Turn to the following pages to compare your answers.
a. high priority? – p. 202
b. appropriate actions for the nurse – p. 203

SECTION 15.2

The supervisor leaves your office to return to his department. You pull Ralph Johnson's health record from your files. As you review the record, you note that three years ago Ralph exhibited similar behavior. He was admitted to an alcohol and drug abuse rehabilitation program for a period of one month. He was referred to Alcoholics Anonymous at the time of discharge. Upon return to the company, Ralph requested a transfer to his present department.

It is now late Tuesday morning. The supervisor stops in your office. He says he had a meeting with Ralph yesterday afternoon and confronted him about the diminished quality of his work, his inconsistent behavior, and the odor of alcohol on his breath. He says Ralph denied having a drinking problem, terminated the conversation, and avoided any contact with him for the rest of the afternoon. He says Ralph arrived early this morning and has been very productive today. However, he is not talking to the supervisor or any of his co-workers. The supervisor says he thinks he acted too quickly in confronting Ralph and perhaps could have helped Ralph in a less direct way.

In the work space provided answer the following questions:

a. Do you think the supervisor's reaction is unusual? Support your answer with rationale.
b. Do you agree with the supervisor that he acted too quickly in confronting Ralph? Support your opinion with rationale.
c. Is it appropriate for you to tell the supervisor about the information you obtained from Ralph's health record? Support your answer with rationale.

Student Work Space

Turn to the following pages to compare your answers.
a. supervisor's reaction – p. 207
b. agree/disagree with the supervisor – p. 208
c. sharing employee information – p. 210

SECTION 15.3

It is now the following Monday morning. Ralph Johnson arrives in your office. He says he has a problem he would like to talk to you about.

In the work space provided:

    a. Identify what specific actions you would take in initiating a therapeutic relationship with Ralph.

    b. Support your approaches with rationale.

Student Work Space

Turn to the following pages to compare your answers.
a. initiating a therapeutic relationship – p. 211
b. rationale – p. 211

SECTION 15.4

Ralph seems nervous as he begins to talk. He says that he knows his supervisor has spoken with you about him. He says he thinks his supervisor might be right. Friday night he was stopped by the state police for DWI (driving while intoxicated) and had to spend the night in jail. He will have to appear in court and does not know what may result from that. You tell him he may be required to pay a fine and attend a special course on the hazards of drunk driving. In response to your statement, Ralph says this is the first time he has been stopped. You tell him that the penalties for successive offenses become more severe; depending on state laws, he could lose his license to drive.

You acknowledge to Ralph that you have reviewed his health record and are aware of his previous problem with alcohol. Ralph says he went to Alcoholics Anonymous a few times but stopped because he was sure he was strong enough to handle the problem himself.

As you investigate stressors in Ralph's life you ask him about his family relationships. He says his family life is "pretty mixed up." Six weeks ago his wife left him because of his drinking; she moved to her parents' home 100 miles away and took both of their children with her. He has seen the children twice since they left. In an attempt to cope with their leaving he has continued to drink.

In the work space provided:

    a. Using your own words, write what you would *say* in your *initial responses* to Ralph when he admits his drinking problem *and* when he discloses to you the problems he is facing.

Student Work Space

Turn to the following page to compare your answers.
a. your initial responses – p. 212

SECTION 15.5

After exploring his options with you, Ralph says he feels as though his world is falling apart; he says he feels all alone and does not think he can make it by himself. He says he thinks he should be admitted to an alcohol and drug abuse rehabilitation program, but he has some questions to ask before he agrees. His questions are:

> "Because this is my second time, will I lose my job?"

> "Will the guys I work with be told why I'm disappearing for a month?"

In the work space provided:

a. Based upon Ralph's questions, what information would you give him?

b. List the nursing action(s) you will take to assist Ralph in beginning his rehabilitation. Support your actions with rationale.

c. Does your role in this situation end here? State your rationale.

Student Work Space

Turn to the following pages to compare your answers.
a. information to answer Ralph's questions – p. 214
b. nursing actions – p. 214
c. does role end? – p. 216

SECTION 15.6

During the next few weeks, the incident with Ralph frequently comes to your mind. You are concerned about several things bearing on Ralph's situation:

1. The supervisor was frustrated because he thought he had taken too long to suspect Ralph's drinking problem.

2. Once the supervisor did recognize the problem he was uncertain how he should handle it.
3. The company policies regarding the employee with a drinking problem were not helpful.

You review the orientation policies/programs for supervisors and find no information on how to handle the employee with a problem of substance abuse. You review the health-related programs started by the previous nurse and find evidence that one workshop on alcohol abuse was provided for supervisors seven years ago. You think that the company should have a more comprehensive approach to employees with alcohol and drug problems.

In the work space provided answer the following:

    a. Is the development of a company-wide, comprehensive approach to alcohol use and abuse an appropriate role for you, or should that responsibility belong to management? State your rationale.
    b. If your answer is no, stop here. If your answer is yes, *briefly* outline how you would begin to approach such a project.

Student Work Space

Turn to the following pages to compare your answers.
a. appropriateness of role – p. 217
b. beginning approach – p. 218

SECTION 15.7

You complete your data base and it reveals the following:

The number of employees currently employed who have a documented problem with alcohol is 38, or 6.3 percent of the total population. Their accident rate is only slightly higher than that of the random sample of employees without a documented alcohol problem.

This percentage is slightly lower than that in the literature you have surveyed.

Your survey of supervisors indicates that 90 percent (18) of the supervisors express a high interest in each of the areas you asked about, i.e., education programs focused on effects of alcohol and drugs, workshops on working effectively with the employee with an alcohol/drug problem, and prevention of alcohol and drug abuse.

Of the employees you surveyed, 60 percent returned their questionnaires. Of those, 75 percent expressed a high degree of interest in education programs focusing on the effects of alcohol and drugs and prevention of alcohol/drug abuse.

Based upon the above data, your assessment is that Cromwell Computer Company has a need for a comprehensive alcohol and drug abuse program.

In the work space provided:

    a. Identify the outcomes that you think would be appropriate for the program.
    b. Briefly outline your plan for developing such a program.
    c. Identify what level(s) of prevention your program will encompass. Support with rationale.

Student Work Space_____

Turn to the following pages to compare your answers.
    a. program outcomes – p. 219
    b. outline of plan – p. 219
    c. levels of prevention – p. 220

ANSWERS TO SECTION 15.1 ───────────

a. Is this situation of high priority? Support your conclusion with rationale.

If you said the situation with this employee is of high priority, your answer is correct. Addressing the situation as soon as possible allows for intervention, prevention of complications (for the individual, the family, and the company), and return of the individual to a productive role within the company (Guida, 1978).

Alcohol abuse is a major problem in American society. Statistics indicate that 7 percent of the adult population (over 18 years of age) have a problem with alcohol (Finley, 1981). But what constitutes a problem? When is an individual an alcoholic? How is alcohol abuse defined? For years researchers have been unable to agree on these questions. Dupont & Basen (1980, p. 138) state that an employee has a problem with drugs or alcohol when his or her use of either substance causes health problems and interferes with work performance. In the U.S. Department of Health and Human Services' Fifth Special Report to the U.S. Congress on Alcohol and Health (1983) new attempts are made to clarify the terms:

> . . . the term "alcohol dependence" is used in preference to the more generic "alcoholism." In addition, a separate category of "alcohol abuse" is added to permit greater differentiation. . . . alcohol dependence is differentiated from alcohol abuse by the presence of tolerance or withdrawal symptoms. Both diagnoses include a pattern of pathological use or impairment in social or occupational functioning due to alcohol (U.S. Department of Health and Human Services, 1983, p. 93).

Whether the individual is "alcohol dependent" or an "alcohol abuser," the results are similar—major problems for the individual, the family, and the employer. In this situation the alcoholic will be defined (Stuart & Sundeen, 1983, p. 458) as any person whose drinking patterns interfere with daily activities and/or impair interpersonal relationships.

The problems alcohol abuse presents to the individual and his or her family can be categorized as follows (Room, 1981):

1. Acute health problems such as gastrointestinal upsets and mental confusion.
2. Chronic health problems such as malnutrition, weight loss, cirrhosis of the liver, and gastrointestinal bleeding.
3. Property damage; injuries from automobile accidents, accidents in the home, and elsewhere; and suicide.
4. Criminal actions and family abuse.
5. Behavioral problems such as public drunkenness and altercations with friends and associates.
6. Default on major social roles—work, school, and family.
7. Altered feelings of self-worth, i.e., demoralization and depression, feelings of worthlessness, and loss of control.

Any one of the problems identified above can be overwhelming to the individual and his or her family. Unfortunately, health professionals often see these individuals and families confronted with not just one but several of these problems.

Although the impact of alcohol abuse on American industry is substantial, the exact cost is not known. A report by the U.S. Department of Health and Human Services (1983, p. 95) estimated that in 1977, the total cost of alcohol abuse to the nation was approximately $50 billion—$26 billion in lost employment and productivity, $17 billion spent on health care, and $7 billion in reparations for property loss and crime. These figures have obviously grown with the dramatic increase in health care costs (U.S. Department of Health and Human Services, 1983, p. 95).

Production is lost when the employee arrives late, leaves early, or is absent (Brown, 1981). One study of alcohol problems in seven railroad companies examined absenteeism in measuring lost production. Findings showed that problem drinkers had almost twice the rate of absenteeism of other workers and that the annual cost to the companies was $3.1 million (U.S. Department of Health and Human Services, 1983, p. 93).

Because judgment, coordination, and reaction time are affected by the consumption of alcohol, employees with an alcohol problem are putting themselves and those with whom they work at risk for accidents. One study suggests that alcoholics are two to three times more likely to be involved in work-related accidents than other employees. Results from other studies have been inconsistent. Thus the true impact of alcohol abuse on work-related accidents has not been clearly determined (U.S. Department of Health and Human Services, 1983, p. 85).

b. Identify appropriate actions by the nurse. Support with rationale.

Actions by the nurse	*Rationale*
1. Provide positive reinforcement for the supervisor's decision to seek assistance.	1. The supervisor realizes that he can no longer handle this situation alone. The nurse should provide him with positive reinforcement for this decision and for his foresight in documenting the employee's behavioral changes. It is also appropriate for the nurse to acknowledge the supervisor's feelings, as it is often difficult for a supervisor to report an employee whatever the precipitating factors are (Hawthorne & Davidson, 1983).
2. Educate the supervisor regarding his role with the employee.	2. Since the supervisor has already stated he does not know what his next step should be, the nurse can outline and discuss an appropriate course of action. An appropriate course of action for the supervisor would be: a. Confront Ralph. b. Present Ralph with his options. c. Refer Ralph to the occupational health service.

The course of action that the nurse can suggest to the supervisor, and its rationale, are as follows:

a. Confront Ralph (Brown, 1981; Sisk, 1981).	a. The employee has to be confronted by management regarding his work performance and behavior to help him understand the seriousness of the situation. This is an appropriate role for the supervisor because he knows the employee, has an established relationship with him, and has documentation of changes in be-

Rationale

havior and work performance (Sisk, 1981). Confrontation by the supervisor should point out the discrepancy between the employee's perceptions of his behavior and the supervisor's perceptions of the employee's behavior (Stuart & Sundeen, 1983).

Confrontation is not an easy role for most people and often results in the expression of anger and hostility (Stuart & Sundeen, 1983). The supervisor may need assistance from the occupational health nurse in determining how to confront the employee so that anger and hostility are less likely to result. For example, the supervisor can confront the employee in one of three ways: he can be aggressive, nonassertive, or assertive.

If the supervisor is *aggressive* in his approach, his statements are likely to be accusatory in nature, i.e., "Your behavior at work is . . . Your work is . . . I think you have a problem." This type of statement is very likely to anger the employee, make him defensive, and result in hostility (Pointer & Lancaster, 1984).

If the supervisor is *nonassertive* in his approach, nothing will be accomplished. He may try to talk to the employee, but it is unlikely that he could be direct enough for the employee to know he is being confronted, i.e., "I think there might be a problem . . . I'm not really sure . . . It seems as though . . ." With this type of approach, the supervisor ends up feeling frustrated and the employee continues with his behavior (Pointer & Lancaster, 1984).

If the supervisor is *assertive* in his approach, the employee will be confronted in a caring but firm fashion that is nonaccusatory in nature, i.e., "I care about you as a friend and co-worker. I have some concerns I think we need to discuss. During the last few months I have observed some changes in your relationships with co-workers and in your attendance at work. Several times in the last three weeks, I've noticed the odor of alcohol on your breath. I think alcohol

Rationale

may be related to the changes I've been seeing in you."

The above statements do not accuse—they state the facts. They also separate the employee from his behavior. The supervisor is letting the employee know he cares about him as an individual; it is the behavior (attendance, difficulty getting along with co-workers, drinking alcohol) that is the problem. With this approach, the supervisor feels more comfortable and relaxed, and the employee is less likely to become defensive or angry (Pointer & Lancaster, 1984).

Having described the approach to use, the occupational health nurse needs to find out whether the supervisor feels able to implement the suggested approach. An offer to role-play the situation, with the nurse assuming the role of the employee, might help the supervisor to gain some confidence with this approach.

b. Present Ralph with his options.

b. The employee should be told his options so that he knows he does have a choice in determining what happens. At this point the employee has two options. He can seek professional assistance through the occupational health service, or he can face disciplinary action such as loss of job (Sisk, 1981).

In presenting Ralph with his options, the positive option should receive the most attention and should be presented first. Hopefully this will help the employee begin to understand that management is concerned with his welfare and there is a reasonable option available to him. If the negative option is presented first, it is likely that the employee will focus only on that option and disregard the positive option altogether.

What does the occupational health service offer the employee? This information is included here so that the supervisor can explain more clearly the options for constructive action available to the employee.

Occupational health services will vary from one workplace to the next. The ser-

Rationale

vices offered will generally focus on treatment, education, and prevention (Sisk, 1981). The occupational health nurse is often the first health care professional with whom the employee comes in contact. It is here that the process of treatment, education, and prevention begins. If the employee is in a state of acute crisis, the nurse will assess the situation, intervene, and stabilize the employee and will then refer him to an appropriate community resource. For example, the nurse may need to collaborate with the employee's physician (with the employee's permission) to arrange for admission to an acute care facility, a detoxification unit, or a rehabilitation unit. If the employee is not in a crisis situation, the nurse may refer him to a community counselor and/or to Alcoholics Anonymous. Within each of these settings, treatment, education, and prevention continue. Once the individual returns to work, the nurse maintains intermittent contact with the employee with a continued focus on education and prevention of relapses. Some companies have an employee assistance program to which employees can be referred. (Guida, 1978)

Employee assistance programs (E.A.P.'s) are designed to assist the employee with problems that may be affecting the ability of the employee to perform acceptably. Problems for which an E.A.P. counselor might see an employee are marital, family, substance abuse, financial, psychological, personal, grief reaction, career, or conflict on the job (Bloomberg, 1984). E.A.P.'s grew out of programs designed in the 1930s and 1940s specifically to help the alcoholic deal with his or her problem and become a more productive employee. Referral to the E.A.P. can come from the employee, a co-worker, family member, friend, occupational health nurse, or the employee's supervisor. The E.A.P. counselor assesses the employee and intervenes as appropriate. A counselor who thinks the employee should be referred beyond the E.A.P. will do so with the employee's permission. Large companies may have E.A.P. coun-

Rationale

selor(s) on the staff; smaller companies may contract for the services of an E.A.P. counselor in private practice in the community (Bloomberg, 1984).

c. Refer Ralph to the occupational health service (Brown, 1981; Sisk, 1981).

c. Monitoring and evaluating the employee's job performance is the supervisor's role. The supervisor should not attempt to counsel the employee. Referral to health care professionals allows the supervisor to remain in his role and transfers the responsibility for counseling, intervention, and follow-up to the health care professionals (Sisk, 1981; Hawthorne & Davidson, 1983).

Actions by the nurse	*Rationale*
3. Intervene with the employee when he responds to the supervisor's referral.	3. The nurse has outlined the appropriate course of action for the supervisor and must now wait until the employee seeks assistance. If the situation should become more acute—e.g., if the employee has an accident or experiences delirium tremens—the nurse may intervene before the course of action by the supervisor is completed.
4. Offer follow-up for the supervisor.	4. The supervisor has an established relationship with the employee. By reporting the employee and confronting him, the supervisor places himself in a difficult position. As a result, he may experience stressors similar to those seen in family members of the alcoholic, i.e., feelings of guilt or failure.

ANSWERS TO SECTION 15.2

a. Is the supervisor's reaction unusual?

The supervisor's reaction is not unusual at all. Dealing with the alcoholic on a daily basis can be a frustrating experience, especially for family and friends. Family members often experience feelings of guilt, failure, and helplessness. Family members tend to feel that they are responsible for the alcoholic's behavior and can help change it. As a result they may make excuses, cover up, and try to avoid any confrontations. At times family members react to the stress the alcohol abuse is having upon them by actually demonstrating behaviors similar to those of the alcoholic, i.e., fatigue, mood changes, irritability, and social withdrawal (Hawthorne & Davidson, 1983).

The employee's supervisor, although not a family member, does have a unique relationship with the individual and interacts with him on a daily basis. Because of this relationship, the supervisor may, in fact, experience some of the same feelings felt by family members. For example, when the employee's productivity decreases, the supervisor may make excuses for him or her. The supervisor may value the employee's friendship on a personal level and, in an attempt to maintain that friendship, avoid confronting the individual about his or her behavior (Hawthorne & Davidson, 1983).

In order to cope with an alcoholic family member some family members seek assistance outside the family through individual or family counseling sessions and through the self-help group Al-Anon.

Unfortunately, the concept of self-help groups is still foreign to many health care professionals. The focus of the self-help group is one of people helping people gain and maintain control over the problems in their lives. Within the group, the individual has a chance to discuss his or her fears, frustrations, etc., with others who can genuinely empathize because they have been confronted with similar problems in their own lives. Participation in the group can bring about increased self-awareness and improved self-esteem. Positive reinforcement from the group is another benefit. With time, the individual develops a new sense of responsibility for his or her behavior (Nix, 1980).

Self-help groups are increasing in number throughout the country. Alcoholics Anonymous, Al-Anon, Overeaters Anonymous, Gamblers Anonymous, and Parents Anonymous are some of the more widely publicized groups.

If you have never attended a self-help group meeting to understand what happens there, perhaps you should! Since some of the meetings may be closed to visitors, a telephone call to the organization is recommended to arrange for an observation.

The supervisor may also need assistance to be able to work effectively with the alcoholic employee. He may benefit from individual counseling services through the occupational health service or through the employee assistance program (if available). He may benefit from attending Al-Anon meetings. The supervisor may also benefit from small group discussions with other supervisors and the occupational health nurse that give him an opportunity to discuss his feelings and frustrations and learn effective ways of working with the alcoholic employee, i.e., how to stop feeling guilty, how to stop covering up for the employee, etc.

b. Do you agree with the supervisor that he acted too quickly in confronting Ralph?

If you agree with the supervisor that perhaps he acted too quickly in confronting Ralph and that he could have helped Ralph in a less direct way, you are *playing the alcoholic's games* in the same way the supervisor is.

Continue reading . . .

If you disagree with the supervisor, you are *correct*. The *active* alcoholic employee (that is, one who is currently abusing alcohol as opposed to a recovering alcoholic who is now abstaining) cannot be ignored. The work site is not the place for the active alcoholic. Decreased productivity is costly for the company. More important, the active alcoholic and those he or she works with are at greater risk for accidents—an even greater loss to the company in terms of workers' compensation and increasing insurance rates. Making excuses for the alcoholic and trying an indirect approach to the problem are not appropriate; direct confrontation is necessary. The supervisor's actions of the previous day were not only appropriate but necessary.

This is a good time for the occupational health nurse to talk with the supervisor about the impact we, as individuals, have on changing another person's behavior.

Can you change someone else's behavior? When you think about this question in a realistic manner, the answer becomes painfully clear: No, you cannot change another person's behavior. Families, friends, and health professionals can confront the individual with his or her behavior, acquaint him or her with the hazards of continuing the behavior, and role-model an alternative behavior. These actions may in the long run influence the individual, but the fact remains: The actual change has to come from within the individual.

Hochbaum, Kegeles, Leventhal, and Rosenstock (Rosenstock, 1974) have developed a framework called the Health Belief Model, which attempts to explain what motivates people to seek ways to prevent illness—in essence to change their behavior. The Health Belief Model (Rosenstock, 1974) theorizes that in order for an individual to perform illness-preventing acts, the individual needs to have three specific perceptions:

1. The individual must *perceive that he or she is susceptible* to a specific disease.
2. The individual must *perceive that contracting the disease would have consequences severe enough to affect his or her life-style.*
3. The individual must *perceive* that the *benefits* derived from the change in behavior *outweigh the barriers* which have, in the past, prevented this change in behavior.

Variables which may affect these perceptions are the individual's age, culture, sex, and educational background. In addition, the Health Belief Model asserts that the individual can be influenced by *cues to action.* Cues to action may be information or an awareness obtained from a friend, health professional, the media, etc.

Let's apply the components of the Health Belief Model to the situation with Ralph. In order for Ralph to perform illness-preventing acts, i.e., change his behavior (give up alcohol), the following need to occur:

1. He must *perceive that he is susceptible* to a specific disease, in this case alcoholism. Unfortunately, Ralph denied to his supervisor that he has a drinking problem. As long as he maintains his denial, his behavior will not change. Denial is common in the alcoholic and is often the major factor standing between the alcoholic and rehabilitation. Denial is often accompanied by statements such as "I can handle it," "I don't have a problem—you do," "I maintain my responsibilities—I go to work every day." How long the denial lasts depends totally on the individual and the life events with which he is faced.
2. He must *perceive that contracting the disease would have consequences severe enough to affect his life-style.* At this time there is no evidence that Ralph understands how his drinking can affect (or already has affected) his life-style. The fact that he has been confronted by the supervisor and given options, i.e., rehabilitation or disciplinary action, may (or may not) help him to understand the seriousness of the situation. For example, the loss of his job is likely to have a severe impact upon his life-style and may be the factor that makes Ralph address his behavior. His perception may well be influenced by his prior experience with this problem.
3. He must *perceive that the benefits* he would derive from changing his behavior *outweigh the barriers* which have, in the past, kept him from changing his behavior. Because Ralph has not been interviewed by the occupational health nurse, it is difficult to determine

what Ralph would see as benefits to not drinking and what "excuses" (barriers) he would give for choosing not to stop. Alcoholics who have stopped drinking identify the following benefits: feeling better, looking better, increased stamina, increased productivity, improved concentration, improved sleep patterns, and more satisfying relationships with family and friends. The "excuses" (barriers) that originally kept them from stopping are: "It will take too much effort," "It's easier to drink," "I like drinking," "I need to drink," "I'm afraid of changing," and—often the key barrier—"I don't have a problem!" In Ralph's situation, his prior experience will be an influencing factor.

In Ralph's situation the *cues to action* that can be identified are the concern of the supervisor and the confrontation by the supervisor. Other cues may occur later or may be occurring within Ralph's family; however, that information is not available at this time. By discussing the above information, the occupational health nurse can help the supervisor understand that he does play an important role with Ralph, but cannot accept responsibility for changing Ralph's behavior; only Ralph can do that. Ralph has to:

1. Believe there is a reason for changing.
2. Want to change because the consequences of his behavior are severely affecting his life-style.
3. Believe that making the change will not be too difficult for him.

c. Is it appropriate for you to tell the supervisor about the information you obtained from Ralph's health record? Support your answer with rationale.

If you said it is appropriate to share the information from Ralph's health record with the supervisor, *your answer is incorrect.* You may have reasoned that sharing the information would help to reassure Ralph's supervisor that his actions of the previous day (confronting Ralph) were appropriate. This is not an appropriate reason. Continue reading to determine under what conditions it is appropriate to share information from an employee health record.

If you said it is not appropriate for the nurse to share the information from Ralph's health record regarding his history of alcohol abuse and rehabilitation, you are correct. Confidentiality in all matters related to employees, including their health records, is essential. Reif (1983, p. 38) states that meaningful communication between the occupational health nurse and the employee can occur only if the employee is assured that the information discussed with the nurse (and recorded in his or her health record) will remain confidential. The employee must also be assured that access to the health record is limited to health professionals within the company, with the following exceptions (Reif, 1983, p. 38):

1. Life-threatening emergencies
2. Authorized release to a personal physician
3. Workers' compensation cases (as mandated by law)
4. Compliance with government regulations

In the situation described, Ralph's supervisor is questioning his actions of the previous day. It could be tempting to the nurse to share her knowledge of Ralph's previous problem with alcohol as a means of reassuring the supervisor that his actions were appropriate; however, reassuring the supervisor does not fall within any of the four exceptions listed above.

ANSWERS TO SECTION 15.3

a. Identify what specific actions you would take in initiating a therapeutic relationship with Ralph.
b. Support your approaches with rationale.

There is no magic formula for initiating a therapeutic relationship with a client. Some nurses are able to do it effectively; others are not. What do those who are effective do? Three things:

1. They care about the client.
2. They understand the impact they can have on a client when they communicate effectively.
3. They use their knowledge of basic communication practices selectively when establishing a nurse-client relationship.

At times, even the most effective nurses will have difficulty initiating a therapeutic relationship with substance abusers. Since conflicting values may play a role, nurses need to examine their own values in relation to substance use and abuse. The nurse needs to be constantly aware of the need to maintain objectivity. It may be appropriate to allow another nurse to intervene (if that's possible). Guida (1978, p. 49) states that there are some nurses who, because of personal characteristics and interests, will be better able to work with substance abusers. Some of these characteristics are:

1. A high tolerance for frustration and the ability to take recurrence and setbacks in stride.
2. The ability to strike a reasonable balance between dependence and independence: the nurse will neither exploit the patient's needs for dependency nor ignore them.
3. The ability to assess realistically what can and cannot be done.

The following actions (some or all) are suggested to initiate a therapeutic relationship with Ralph. How they are used and the order in which they are used will naturally vary with each nurse.

a. Initiating a therapeutic relationship	b. Rationale
1. Provide privacy.	1. Closing the health office door or moving into a private section of the office lets Ralph know you value and respect him and what he has to say.
2. Help Ralph to feel comfortable.	2. Sit down with him so you are both at the same eye level; sit close to him without a desk or table between you. Avoid standing and "looking down" at Ralph while he is sitting.
3. Shake hands with Ralph (Stuart & Sundeen, 1983).	3. Touching shows acceptance of the employee by the nurse. A simple handshake conveys that acceptance.
4. Clarify the purpose of	4. In this situation Ralph has come to you indicating he thinks he has a problem.

a. Initiating a therapeutic relationship	*b. Rationale*
the meeting (Stuart & Sundeen, 1983).	Help him to identify as clearly as possible what he thinks is his problem.
5. Respond with genuineness (Stuart & Sundeen, 1983).	5. If Ralph senses that you are sincere in wanting to help him, he will probably feel more comfortable in being open and honest with you. If your values are in conflict with the client's behavior, i.e., substance abuse, you'll need to try to maintain objectivity. If objectivity is not maintained, the difference in values will emerge and the client may pull away from you.
6. Confront Ralph with his behavior (Stuart & Sundeen, 1983).	6. Assertive confrontation by you regarding his behavior reaffirms to the employee that he does, indeed, have a problem with alcohol.
7. Ask Ralph what he sees as his options for dealing with his problems.	7. A client will more readily follow a plan that he or she has developed. Having previously coped with this problem, Ralph will know some of his options. The role of the nurse in this part of the interaction is to acknowledge the options that the client suggests, to help to evaluate the advantages and disadvantages of each one, to suggest options that may have been omitted, and to resist the natural inclination to rush Ralph's decision. Encourage Ralph to think about his options, to discuss them with his family and any others he feels could be helpful, and to return for another appointment with you in a few days.
8. Support his decision to seek help.	8. Provide him with positive reinforcement for taking positive steps to change behavior patterns that have been disruptive to him and his family.

ANSWERS TO SECTION 15.4

a. Your initial responses.

The following would be appropriate as an initial response by the nurse when Ralph admits he has a drinking problem.

"It sounds as though this has been a difficult week for you."

"It must have taken a great deal of courage to come here this morning."

"I'm glad you're here. It must have been difficult for you to come."

The following would be appropriate as an initial response by the nurse to Ralph's disclosures about his being stopped by the state police and his family problems.

"This must be a difficult time for you."

"It sounds as though the past few months have been difficult for you. Would you like to tell me about it?"

"It sounds as though you're facing several major problems."

Your responses to Ralph should be ones that will facilitate therapeutic communication between the occupational health nurse and the employee. The initial response needs to convey:

1. *Acknowledgment* of the employee's concerns.
2. *Respect* for the employee (Stuart & Sundeen, 1983).
3. *Empathy* regarding the employee's concerns (Stuart & Sundeen, 1983).
4. *Reassurance* that the employee's concerns will be addressed.

Acknowledgment of the employee's concerns conveys to the employee that the nurse is really hearing what the employee is saying. Acknowledgment by the nurse needs to be accepting and nonjudgmental in nature. If Ralph thinks his behavior is being judged by the nurse, he will not communicate openly.

Respect (Stuart & Sundeen, 1983) – valuing the employee as an individual. The employee's values, culture, beliefs, behaviors, etc., may differ substantially from those of the nurse. A judgmental or condescending approach to the employee by the nurse communicates to the employee that what he thinks and feels are viewed as unimportant. The nurse can demonstrate respect for Ralph by acknowledging that he has taken the difficult first step of seeking help with his drinking problem and by showing a sincere interest in helping him. Ralph has come willingly to seek assistance from the occupational health nurse. This action has very likely taken a great deal of effort on his part. Acknowledging his action conveys to him your respect for him as an individual.

Empathy (Stuart & Sundeen, 1983) – allowing oneself to feel what the client is feeling. Realistically, the individual nurse may not be able to feel what the client is feeling through personal experience. However, the nurse may have worked with other alcoholics and observed the pain and frustration they encountered in facing their drinking problem. Placing yourself in Ralph's shoes helps you understand better what he has been experiencing. However, it is also important to remain objective. Remember that Ralph's current problems are the result of his own health-damaging behavior.

Reassurance that the employee's concerns can and will be addressed can be beneficial in reducing stress in the employee. Reassurance should be sincere and genuine; it should not be patronizing in nature. In this situation letting the employee know that he has come to the appropriate place to seek assistance can help to reassure him that he is no longer facing his problem(s) alone.

Look at the responses you have written. Do your responses convey acknowledgment, respect, empathy, and reassurance? If they do, congratulations! If they don't, what is missing? How can you make your responses more effective?

ANSWERS TO SECTION 15.5

a. Information to answer Ralph's questions.

Will Ralph lose his job because it's the second time he has experienced a problem with alcohol?

In most companies, the policy is that Ralph will not lose his job as long as he obtains professional help (either through individual/family counseling or admission to an alcohol and drug abuse program) and follows through with the recommendations, such as continued counseling and attendance at Alcoholics Anonymous meetings.

Ralph needs to understand that even though this is the second time his drinking has caused problems at work, it is not a discriminating factor. You can reinforce to him that alcoholism is an addiction to a very powerful drug; it is an illness. As with any other illness, treatment, education, and prevention of related problems will help the individual to return to his optimum level of functioning.

Ralph also needs to understand that he will be expected to assume responsibility for controlling his alcohol problem and preventing related problems when he returns to work. One of the most successful programs, worldwide, that helps alcoholics accept and maintain responsibility for their behavior and prevent alcohol-related problems is Alcoholics Anonymous. Through Alcoholics Anonymous alcoholics find the courage to face each day without alcohol, learning to depend on themselves and the support of others rather than alcohol. The amount of support an individual may need from A.A. varies with the individual. For example, some may attend A.A. meetings several times a week, others may attend daily, and some may attend more than once a day.

Will Ralph's co-workers be told why he will be away from work?

Ralph needs to be reassured that you, the occupational health nurse, will not be discussing Ralph's medical problems with his co-workers because of the confidential relationship between employee and nurse. Encourage Ralph to assume the responsibility for telling his supervisor. You can remind Ralph that it was because of the supervisor's concern that he was confronted about his behavior changes. It would also be appropriate to encourage Ralph to talk with his co-workers. If Ralph tells his co-workers that he has a problem with alcohol and he will be going to a rehabilitation center, he helps dispel workplace "gossip." Facing his co-workers before he leaves will make his return in a month more comfortable for him and his co-workers.

b. Nursing actions and rationale.

The following nursing actions would be appropriate in helping Ralph begin his rehabilitation process.

a. Nursing actions	*b. Rationale*
1. Acknowledge Ralph's concerns and answer his questions.	1. If Ralph feels the nurse views his concerns as valid, it is likely he will share additional concerns. If the nurse pays little attention to what the employee is asking or dismisses the concerns as insignificant, the employee may lose trust in the employee-nurse relationship.
2. Encourage Ralph to take his time making his decision.	2. Ralph is more likely to make a firm decision if he takes a few days to think about it and to discuss his options with friends and family members.
3. Provide Ralph with positive reinforcement that he has made a difficult but positive decision.	3. Responding to Ralph's decision in a positive fashion indicates to him that the nurse *empathizes* with him regarding the difficulty of making such a decision and *respects* his decision (Stuart & Sundeen, 1983).
4. Contact the physician to refer Ralph for treatment.	4. In the majority of situations, admission to a residential alcohol and drug abuse program is based on a referral by a physician. Give Ralph the option of deciding whether he wants his personal physician or the company physician to make the referral. Before making the actual referral, the physician may want to evaluate the employee's physical status in order to: a. Assess the employee's known medical problems. b. Assess any new medical problems. c. Determine whether the employee needs detoxification upon admission. d. Determine, if medical problems exist, whether the employee's health status can tolerate a detoxification process. Admission to a residential treatment program may be possible immediately or may take several days to arrange.
5. Help Ralph identify a support system to help him until his admission.	5. If admission to a residential treatment program cannot be arranged immediately, Ralph will need an effective support system to depend on so that he does not return to his behavior of depending on alcohol. An effective support system will be able to provide him with moral support and company at home or en route to the residential alcohol and drug abuse program.

a. Nursing actions	*b. Rationale*
	Friends, family, or co-workers can be an effective support system. With the nurse's assistance, Ralph may be able to identify his support system. Because Ralph is separated from his wife and children, he may (or may not) feel that friends and other family members would be more supportive at this time (Finley, 1981).
	Another source of support would be people Ralph knew when he previously belonged to Alcoholics Anonymous. Members respond readily and immediately to any individual who asks for help. There may be A.A. members within the company who, if contacted by Ralph or the occupational health nurse (with Ralph's permission), would provide the support system Ralph needs until he is admitted to the residential alcohol and drug abuse program.

If you were able to identify most (or all) of the above actions and rationale, congratulations! If you were not, take a second look at those that are missing from your list and review the supporting rationale.

c. Does your role in this situation end here? State your rationale.

If you think that your role does not end here, you are correct. Your role will continue once Ralph returns to the company. Before returning to work, any employee who has been on an extended medical leave from the company needs to contact the occupational health service. He will need physician approval to return to work; updated medical information regarding his problem, progress, and activity restrictions; and recommendations for follow-up.

Based upon the above information, this is an appropriate time for the occupational health nurse to discuss with the employee his plans for following through with the recommendations. For example, if counseling was recommended, has he seen the counselor? Has he made an appointment? If Alcoholics Anonymous was recommended, has he started attending meetings? How will he fit the meetings into his workday?

This initial interview with the employee upon his return is also an appropriate time to discuss the employee's perception of other personal/family problems with which he is confronted. This gives the nurse the opportunity to assess how the employee is coping with other personal/family problems and to convey to the employee that the total welfare of the employee is of concern to the nurse and the company. To maintain contact with the employee, the nurse should encourage the employee to schedule an appointment for a follow-up visit before he leaves the occupational health office.

ANSWERS TO SECTION 15.6 ————————

a. Is the development of a company-wide, comprehensive approach to alcohol use and abuse an appropriate role for the occupational health nurse?

If you answered yes, congratulations! You are correct. The profound effects alcohol abuse has on individual employees, their families, and the company have been discussed earlier. It is unlikely that Ralph Johnson is the only employee within the company who has/will have a problem with alcohol. Using the statistics discussed earlier, it is conceivable that 7 percent, or 42 of the company's 600 employees, could have a problem with alcohol.

A comprehensive approach to alcohol use and abuse by the company is not only appropriate; it is a necessity. Early diagnosis and early intervention could prevent many problems for the employee, the family, and the company. The individual could be identified sooner, counseled into treatment sooner, and return to family life and the work force at a higher level of functioning sooner.

But is the individual problem drinker the only focus in a comprehensive approach to alcohol use and abuse by the company? Certainly the individual (as shown by this situation) is a priority. However, the following *populations* or *aggregates* need to be considered:

1. All company employees
2. The subpopulation of individuals who have/have had a problem with alcohol

Williams (1984, p. 809) defines *population* as a collection of individuals who share one or more personal or environmental characteristics. (The same definition has been applied to the term *aggregate* [Williams, 1977]). Both groups identified above meet the definition of a population or an aggregate as follows:

	Characteristics	
Population (Aggregate)	*Personal*	*Environmental*
All company employees	1. Adults	1. Work in the same environment
Subpopulation of employees	1. Adults 2. Have a problem with alcohol	1. Work in the same environment

As a community health nurse, the occupational health nurse has an opportunity to move beyond the individual and family as client to the broader context of population-focused nursing, with the community as client. Population-focused nursing is the primary factor that makes community health nursing a specialty. The purpose of population-focused practice is to help the population (aggregate) achieve a higher level of wellness through primary, secondary, and/or tertiary prevention.

Unfortunately, the majority of community health nurses employed at the staff level do not have an opportunity to plan for and practice population-focused nursing. The responsibility for population-focused practice generally falls at the administrative or supervisory level. As a result the staff nurse does not have a clear understanding of how to work effectively with aggregates. (Williams, 1984)

In this situation the occupational health nurse has a unique opportunity to investigate further and, based upon the findings, make a choice to continue with the status quo or to accept the responsibility of practicing population-focused nursing.

b. *Briefly* outline how you would begin to approach such a project.

In population-focused practice, as in nursing care of the individual and the family, plans cannot be made and implemented on the basis of intuition or previous experience alone. A comprehensive data base is needed to make an accurate needs assessment (Chenoweth, 1984; Stanhope & Lee, 1984). Both objective and subjective data should be gathered.

Objective data

1. Review the literature to gather national statistics on alcohol abuse similar to those discussed in the early sections of this Situation. Document all sources.
2. Review employee health records to determine the number of employees having documented problems with alcohol (Chenoweth, 1984; Lukes, 1984). From these records calculate the number of workdays lost and the number of accidents in which these employees were involved in the workplace.
3. Review a random sample of employee health records of individuals who do not have a documented problem with alcohol; calculate the same data.
4. Compare the two groups of employee health records; compare the findings with national statistics.

Before gathering subjective data, schedule a meeting with your immediate supervisor to determine who in administration should be contacted. Then schedule a meeting with the appropriate administrative personnel. Let them know of your concerns and present the objective data you have gathered. Remember to present the comparisons outlined above, i.e., employees with a documented drinking problem compared with other employees, and both groups compared with the national statistics you've gathered. For your statistics to mean anything to the administration you must be able to compare them with similar statistics (Gutmann, 1976) and project them on the work population in the company.

One of your primary reasons for meeting with the company administrators is to inform them of present and potential problems and obtain their support and participation in the project (Douglass & Bevis, 1983). The best-laid plans can be sabotaged by administrators if the lines of communication are not kept open and administrative support is not obtained.

Subjective data (Chenoweth, 1984)

1. Survey the company supervisors to determine what their needs are in terms of alcohol awareness, working with the alcoholic employee, and prevention.
2. Survey the employees to determine what their needs are in terms of alcohol awareness and prevention as a personal as well as family problem.

ANSWERS TO SECTION 15.7

a. Outcomes appropriate for the program.

The following outcomes would be appropriate for a comprehensive alcohol and drug abuse program within the company (Lukes, 1984):

1. Supervisors will be able to identify and confront employees with alcohol and/or drug abuse problems.
2. Employees with alcohol and/or drug abuse problems will receive prompt treatment.
3. Employees with alcohol and/or drug abuse problems will be able to return to their jobs and maintain satisfactory performance and attendance records.
4. Employees will be able to identify the role Alcoholics Anonymous plays in rehabilitating individuals with alcohol problems.
5. Employees with alcohol and/or drug abuse problems will be offered the opportunity to use a company conference room, on their own time, to meet regularly as a group under the auspices of Alcoholics Anonymous to maintain their optimum level of functioning.
6. Employees will be able to identify physiological and psychosocial effects of alcohol and drug abuse.
7. Employees will be able to identify effective ways of preventing alcohol and/or drug abuse.
8. Policies describing the roles of the company and the occupational health service in working with employees with alcohol and drug problems will be clearly defined.
9. Company management will support the development and implementation of a comprehensive alcohol and drug abuse program for employees by the occupational health service.

If you identified outcomes similar to many or all of the above, good job! If you did not, take this opportunity to review yours to determine what's missing. Outcomes should be written to include employees with alcohol and/or drug problems, employees without alcohol and/or drug problems, supervisors, and management, and they should be expressed in behavioral terms so that the results can be evaluated.

If the outcomes you identified are more specific than those listed above, perhaps they belong under one of the identified outcomes as a means of achieving the outcome.

b. Briefly outline your plan for developing your program.

Assessment: Refer to answers section 15.6b if you have any questions about how the assessment was made.

Plan:

1. Contact the company physician and company management to present the findings of your needs assessment. Maintain open communication with the physician and company management at all times to facilitate the interpersonal exchanges necessary for planned change to occur (Douglass & Bevis, 1983).

2. Invite the physician, representatives of management, the supervisory group, and employees to participate in the planning (Douglass & Bevis, 1983; Reinertsen, 1983).
3. Identify the desired outcomes.
4. Examine resources available within the company. An excellent program may never be implemented if the resources are unavailable.
5. Examine resources available outside the company, i.e., monetary and/or personnel. Monetary resources could include community, state, and federal grant monies; personnel resources may include counselors, health educators, and self-help groups.
6. Approach one aspect of your program at a time. Establish where you and those working with you (physician and management) would like to begin, i.e., identification of employees with alcohol problems, policies, treatment, or prevention. Where you begin can be influenced by a great number of factors; each situation has to be carefully assessed by those involved in the planning process. For example, one group of planners may elect to begin with writing policies for how the employee with an alcohol or drug problem will be handled; another group may elect to begin with workshops for supervisors. No one planning process is right for all organizations.
7. Once you have established your priorities, outline step by step how you will achieve the outcome(s).
8. Implement the step-by-step plan (Chenoweth, 1984). For example, if the focus is prevention/education, specific steps might be to outline the content to be covered, obtain resources needed (e.g., outside speakers), etc.
9. Evaluate intermittently to determine effectiveness. Make changes as needed and reevaluate the process.

Program development does not take place overnight. Thoughtful planning takes time.

c. What levels of prevention your program will encompass.

If you think a comprehensive alcohol and drug abuse program should encompass all three levels of prevention, you are correct. In this setting, there are employees who individually or in their families already have a documented alcohol and/or drug problem, employees who may develop a problem in the future, and employees who do not have a problem with alcohol and/or drugs and with further education may be able to prevent such problems.

Levels of prevention

Tertiary. Shamansky and Clausen (1980, p. 106) state: Tertiary prevention occurs "when a defect or disability is fixed, stabilized, or irreversible. Rehabilitation, the goal of tertiary prevention, is more than halting the disease process itself; it is restoring the individual to an optimum level of function within the constraints of the disability." The company employees who have a documented alcohol and/or drug problem are indeed in a period of rehabilitation that will continue for the rest of their lives. Giving these employees the opportunity to meet as members of Alcoholics Anonymous using company facilities at lunchtime or immediately following work helps them to understand that the company values them as individuals and is encouraging them to continue with their rehabilitative process.

Secondary. Shamansky and Clausen (1980, p. 106) state: "Secondary prevention emphasizes early diagnosis and prompt intervention to halt the pathological process, thereby shortening its duration and severity and enabling the individual to regain normal function at the earliest possible point. Early diagnosis is illustrated by use of a comprehensive nursing assessment, which may reveal the need for further medical evaluation." Early intervention and prompt treatment are included in the desired outcomes for this program. Any employee may fall into this category, i.e., the rehabilitated employee who suddenly resumes his or her alcohol and/or drug abuse or the person who begins to demonstrate behaviors indicative of an alcohol and/or drug problem. Offering workshops designed to help supervisors recognize behavior changes indicative of alcohol and/or drug abuse is clearly secondary prevention.

Primary. Last, but by no means least, is primary prevention. Shamansky and Clausen (1980, p. 106) state: "Primary prevention is prevention in the true sense of the word; it precedes disease or dysfunction and is applied to a generally healthy population. The targets are those individuals considered physically or emotionally healthy and exhibiting normal or maximum functioning. Primary prevention is not therapeutic; it does not consist of symptom identification and use of therapeutic skills. Primary prevention includes generalized health promotion as well as protection against a specific disease."

A comprehensive alcohol and drug abuse program needs to include both specific disease prevention and health promotion. Employees who do not have an alcohol and/or drug problem need to know specifically how to prevent such a problem from developing. In addition, there needs to be a focus on health promotion: helping individuals to feel good about themselves and to continue to make positive health-generating choices for themselves and their families.

Resolution

Ralph Johnson was admitted to a residential treatment facility for alcohol and drug abusers; he remained at the facility for one month. Upon discharge Ralph returned to the company, working half-days for two weeks. During those initial weeks, he attended Alcoholics Anonymous meetings daily. When he returned to work full-time he continued to attend A.A. meetings four times a week. Ralph received individual counseling for approximately six months. Ralph's wife and children returned home two months after his discharge; Ralph and his wife are at present going to a marriage counselor.

Cromwell Computer Company administrators supported the concept of developing a comprehensive alcohol and drug abuse program. Policies outlining the company's philosophy on helping the employee with an alcohol and/or drug problem are in place and working well. The process for helping the employee with a problem has been strengthened in all areas: workshops for supervisors were held, and the few employees who have been processed received treatment promptly. A daily meeting of Alcoholics Anonymous is held at lunchtime in a private section of the employee cafeteria. In addition, a counselor was hired to work with the occupational health nurse in counseling these employees. It was reported to the occupational health nurse that several employees who have not had an abuse problem while working for Cromwell are attending the A.A. meetings.

Future company plans are expansion of the counseling services offered by establishing an employee assistance program. Community-based counselors will work closely with the company and see employees through self-referral or referral from the occupational health nurse.

References

Bloomberg, G. (1984). E.A.P. comes of age in the workplace. *Vermont Registered Nurse,* June, 7–8.

Brown, M. L. (1981). *Occupational health nursing.* New York: Springer.

Chenoweth, D. (1984). Shaping up health promotion for introduction into a workplace. *Occupational Health and Safety* 32(6): 49–54.

Douglass, L. M., & Bevis, E. D. (1983). *Nursing management and leadership in action.* St. Louis: Mosby.

Dupont, R. L., & Basen, M. M. (1980). Control of alcohol and drug abuse in industry—a literature review. *Public Health Reports* 95(2):137–148.

Finley, B. (1981). Counseling the alcoholic client. *Journal of Psychiatric Nursing and Mental Health Services* 19(6):33–34.

Guida, M. A. (1978). Occupational health nurses are in the best position to help workers fight alcoholism. *Occupational Health and Safety* 47(5):48–52.

Gutmann, K. (1976). Community assessment. Lecture. Chestnut Hill, MA: Boston College.

Hawthorne, W. B., & Davidson, B. N. (1983). The alcoholic's supervisor: Another victim in need. *Occupational Health and Safety* 52(9):28–29, 40.

Lukes, E. (1984). The nursing process and program planning. *Occupational Health Nursing* 32(5):255–256.

Nix, H. (1980). Why parents anonymous? *Journal of Psychiatric Nursing and Mental Health Services* 18:23–28.

Pointer, P., & Lancaster, J. (1984). Assertiveness in community health nursing. In M. Stanhope & J. Lancaster (Eds.). *Community health nursing.* St. Louis: Mosby (pp. 824–842).

Reif, L. (1983). Access to employee medical records. *Occupational Health Nursing* 31(5):38–40.

Reinertsen, J. (1983). Promoting health is good business. *Occupational Health and Safety* 31(6):18–22.

Room, R. (1981). The case for a problem prevention approach to alcohol, drug and mental problems. *Public Health Reports* 96(1):26–32.

Rosenstock, I. M. (1974). Historical origins of the health belief model. In M. Becker (Ed.). *The health belief model and personal health behavior.* Thorofare, NJ: Slack (pp. 1–8).

Shamansky, S. L., & Clausen, C. L. (1980). Levels of prevention: Examination of the concept. *Nursing Outlook* 28(2):104–108.

Sisk, B. A. (1981). Nursing roles in alcoholism: The employee assistance program in a one-nurse setting. *Occupational Health Nursing* 29(3):9–13.

Stanhope, M., & Lee, G. (1984). Program planning and evaluation in community health. In M. Stanhope & J. Lancaster (Eds.). *Community health nursing.* St. Louis: Mosby (pp. 201–218).

Stuart, G. W., & Sundeen, S. J. (1983). *Principles and practice of psychiatric nursing.* (2d ed.) St. Louis: Mosby.

U.S. Department of Health and Human Services (1984). *Fifth special report to the U.S. Congress on alcohol and health.* National Institute on Alcohol Abuse and Alcoholism. Rockville, MD: Government Printing Office.

Williams, C. (1977). Community health nursing: What is it? *Nursing Outlook* 25(4): 250–254.

Williams, C. (1984). Population-focused practice. In M. Stanhope & J. Lancaster (Eds.). *Community health nursing.* St. Louis: Mosby (pp. 805–815).

INDEX